The MRCP part 1:
*a system based tutorial*

# The MRCP part 1:
## a system based tutorial

**C.A. O'Callaghan** BM, BCh, MA, MRCP

CLINICAL LECTURER
Molecular Immunology Group
Nuffield Department of Medicine
University of Oxford Institute of Molecular Medicine
John Radcliffe Hospital
Oxford

*b*

Blackwell
Science

© 1997 by
Blackwell Science Ltd
Editorial Offices:
Osney Mead, Oxford OX2 0EL
25 John Street, London WC1N 2BL
23 Ainslie Place, Edinburgh EH3 6AJ
350 Main Street, Malden
 MA 02148 5018, USA
54 University Street, Carlton
 Victoria 3053, Australia

Other Editorial Offices:
Blackwell Wissenschafts-Verlag GmbH
Kurfürstendamm 57
10707 Berlin, Germany

Blackwell Science KK
MG Kodenmacho Building
7–10 Kodenmacho Nihombashi
Chuo-ku, Tokyo 104, Japan

All rights reserved. No part of
this publication may be reproduced,
stored in a retrieval system, or
transmitted, in any form or by any
means, electronic, mechanical,
photocopying, recording or
otherwise, except as permitted by
the UK Copyright, Designs and
Patents Act 1988, without the prior
permission of the copyright owner.

First published 1997

Set by Setrite Typsetters, Hong Kong
Printed and bound in Great Britain
by Hartnolls Ltd, Bodmin, Cornwall

The Blackwell Science logo is a
trade mark of Blackwell Science Ltd,
registered at the United Kingdom
Trade Marks Registry

DISTRIBUTORS

 Marston Book Services Ltd
 PO Box 269
 Abingdon, Oxon OX14 4YN
 (*Orders:* Tel: 01235 465500
  Fax: 01235 465555)

USA
 Blackwell Science, Inc.
 Commerce Place
 350 Main Street
 Malden, MA 02148 5018
 (*Orders:* Tel: 800 759 6102
   617 388 8250
   Fax: 617 388 8255)

Canada
 Copp Clark Professional
 200 Adelaide St, West, 3rd Floor
 Toronto, Ontario M5H 1W7
 (*Orders*: Tel: 416 597-1616
   800 815-9417
   Fax: 416 597-1617)

Australia
 Blackwell Science Pty Ltd
 54 University Street
 Carlton, Victoria 3053
 (*Orders*: Tel: 3 9347 0300
   Fax: 3 9347 5001)

A catalogue record for this title
is available from the British Library

ISBN 0-63204-781-X

# Contents

Preface, vii

Examination technique and preparation, 1

## Questions
Cardiology, 15
Endocrinology, 20
Gastroenterology, 25
Haematology, 30
Infection, 34
Nephrology, 39
Neurology, 43
Pharmacology, 48
Respiratory, 53
Rheumatology, 58
Mathematical medicine, 62

## Answers
Cardiology, 69
Endocrinology, 83
Gastroenterology, 93
Haematology, 104
Infection, 114
Nephrology, 124
Neurology, 134
Pharmacology, 146
Respiratory, 157
Rheumatology, 165
Mathematical medicine, 173

Index, 187

# Preface

This book has evolved out of formal and informal teaching that I have been doing over a number of years. The questions have been designed to prepare candidates for the examination in a number of different ways. In the first place, the question topics have been selected to represent material used in the actual examination, and to provide realistic practice for it. This is the product of extensive discussion with candidates over several years. Secondly, the questions have been designed to teach key aspects of core topics which frequently occur in the examination. In line with this, I have tried to provide instructive answers that should not only explain the question but also teach the subject under consideration and so minimize the need for reference to textbooks. In addition, certain new topics have been incorporated which could appear in the examination over the next few years. Thirdly, modern basic and molecular science has been fully integrated with the relevant clinical topics throughout the book, in line with the new style examination.

My aim is to keep this book in touch with the examination and, to this end, I am keen to hear from any candidate about new topics appearing in the examination. If you would like to send questions which you encountered in the examination to me, then that would help future candidates immensely. I would also be delighted to have feedback on this book and suggestions for future editions. Any correspondence can be addressed to me at the publishers office.

I wish all those who are taking the examination good luck and I hope that this book is of some help in preparing for it. Lastly, I would like to thank my family and friends for their support and

## Preface

all those colleagues, junior and senior who have taught me medicine and science.

C.A. O'Callaghan

Oxford 1997

# Examination technique and preparation

The key fact to remember about the MRCP Part 1 examination is that most people who need to pass it do so eventually. However, most candidates wisely want to get it out of the way as soon as possible so that they can tackle the Part 2 examination and move on with their careers. In practice, the main problem facing Part 1 candidates is knowing how best to prepare for the examination. Obviously, if you find that you have enough time, then it can be profitable to do some general background reading, but the most useful preparation is undoubtedly to attempt a good number of well constructed multiple choice questions. Nevertheless, even if you are close to the examination date, it can still pay to do some general preparation by reviewing a few of the key topics which are likely to be examined. After this, or straight away if you are short of time, move on to specific examination preparation, which is attempting practice questions. I have outlined an approach to general and specific preparation below.

## General preparation

The scope of the subject material for the examination is so vast that learning it all from textbooks in the time available is out of the question. The best approach is to focus on the topics that are most likely to come up in the examination. In particular, there are certain topics which are especially suitable for questions of the multiple choice format.

There are several ways of predicting which topics are most likely to come up in the examination. Remember, in the first place, who sets the examination paper. The examiners are usually senior consultant fellows of the royal colleges who are drawn from both the academic sector and the National Health

Service clinical sector. They include fellows working in teaching hospitals and those in district general hospitals, so expect contributions reflecting the interests and approaches of these different groups. Secondly, consider what subjects are currently topical as these are likely to be as fresh in the examiners' minds as in your own. Thirdly, consider what topics are of such central importance in medicine that the examiners feel an obligation to ensure that they appear regularly in the examination. Fourthly, bear in mind those topics which are clearly old favourites with the examiners. Often this is for no particularly obvious reason, other than that they make good multiple choice questions – at least in the minds of the examiners. An example of such an 'old chestnut' would be renal tubular acidosis. Fifthly, try to think what questions an innovative examiner might be proud to have set and had accepted into the examination.

*Predicting examination questions*
1 What interests the examiners?
2 Topical issues.
3 Core medical subjects.
4 Old favourites.
5 Innovative questions.

**Topical subjects**
Topical subjects are relatively easy to spot. For the most part, they will be subjects which have recently been featured in editorials in the major medical journals such as the *New England Journal of Medicine*, *The Lancet* and the *British Medical Journal*. It is certainly well worth spending a few hours in a library glancing over the last year or so of these journals as well as the *Journal of the Royal College of Physicians* and the *Quarterly Journal of Medicine*. Any such topics which you feel are likely to be suitable for questions are worth reading about, always bearing in mind what could be asked in multiple choice format. In addition, any topic which has reached the general media is worth reviewing.

Examination technique and preparation

For example, if there has been an outbreak of meningitis or necrotising fasciitis, it would be foolish not to be well informed about these subjects. As the questions can be compiled several months in advance of the examination date, be particularly alert for what is topical at that time. It is also worth looking at recent copies of the *Journal of the Royal College of Physicians*, to check that there have not been any recent changes to the examination regulations, or the nature of the subject content.

**Core subjects**
There are certain core topics which can never be ignored. Most important are the medical emergencies. These are listed in Table 1 and can often lead to relatively straightforward questions. In any case, they are important in their own right, so ignorance is basically unacceptable and the examiners know this. Again, think how these topics may be examined in multiple choice, true–false format.

**Table 1** Core subjects.

| | |
|---|---|
| Myocardial infarction | Septic arthritis |
| Cardiac arrest | Acute poisoning |
| Gastrointestinal bleeding | Diabetic ketoacidosis |
| Acute epilepsy/Status epilepticus | Pulmonary oedema |
| Acute stroke | Coma |
| Meningitis | Pulmonary embolism |
| Basic arrhythmias | Acute asthma |
| Acute pneumonia | Sickle cell crisis |
| Acute pancreatitis | Acute renal failure |

**Examination favourites**
Old favourites are not difficult to spot. The Royal Colleges have published some of their past papers and it is mandatory that you get these and do all the questions, thinking carefully about how they are constructed and paying careful attention to the topics which come up. In addition to this, try to talk to people

who have sat the examination within the last few years as they may remember questions which occurred in their examination which they had themselves heard of before. Some questions do seem to recur quite frequently. Some of these topics are listed in Table 2. One of the main features of these topics is that they can easily be made into questions with multiple responses following on from a single stem statement.

**Table 2** Favourite subjects.

Renal tubular acidosis
Hyperlipidaemia
Glycogen storage diseases
Hyper- and hypo-parathyroidism
Multiple endocrine neoplasia syndromes
Warfarin interaction
Glucose-6-phosphate dehydrogenase deficiency drug problems
Aspirin overdose
Pregnancy and drugs
Porphyria
Intestinal worms
Vitamin B deficiencies
Aspergillus related respiratory disease
Pulmonary fibrosis and its associates
Causes of standard laboratory test abnormalities

## Innovative questions

Over the last few years, the Royal College has formally announced its intention to increase the basic science content of the examination. They have, however, stated that this will be relevant to the training of junior doctors. The result has been a clear increase in innovative or modern questions. In particular, there have been questions on our current understanding of the molecular biology of disease and the use of molecular biological approaches in the diagnosis and treatment of disease. For those unfamiliar with this type of science, it may seem a daunting prospect to have to learn this material as well as all that was previously required. However, in practice, the questions have been relatively straightforward and predictable. For this reason, a few hours spent on the basics of molecular biology is likely to pay a good dividend. Table 3 lists a few key topics, but it is not necessary to study these topics in great detail. Good sources of information include short undergraduate textbooks on biochemistry, genetics, immunology and basic molecular biology.

**Table 3** Molecular biology.

The genetic basis for disease
  monogenic disorders and the different ways single mutations can cause disease
  polygenic disorders

The distinction between knowing the chromosomal locus for a disease gene and identifying the gene itself

HLA associations

Genetic factors in the infectious pathogens and their role in virulence

Diagnostic methods
  restriction fragment length polymorphism (RFLP)
  sequence analysis
  amplification refractory mutation system (ARMS)
  single stranded conformational polymorphism (SSCP)
  polymerase chain reaction (PCR)
  enzyme linked immunoassay (ELISA)

Therapeutic interventions
  monoclonal antibodies
  cytokine based treatment strategies
  therapy with genetically modified cells
  rational drug design

Examination technique and preparation

## Specific preparation

Whether or not you have been able to do some general preparation as outlined above, you should move on to specific preparation at least 8–12 weeks before the examination. The best way to do this is to attempt a reasonable number of multiple choice questions (MCQs).

### Answering negatively marked MCQs

The reason for doing lots of practice questions is both to learn from the subject content of the questions and to improve your examination technique. The papers are negatively marked which means that you score one mark for a correct answer, that you lose one mark for an incorrect answer and that you score nothing if you do not answer a question. There is undoubtedly a skill to answering negatively marked papers, which lies in being able to determine how sure you are of the answer. Obviously, if you are sure of an answer there is no problem. However, if you are not quite sure then the safe thing to do is to leave the question blank. Doing lots of questions will eventually give you a good feeling for how brave you can afford to be when answering. Always look quite closely at the answers and see whether you would have been better not answering a question, or on the other hand, whether you would have been better following your hunch and answering. In general a fairly cautious approach is best at first.

Under no circumstances be tempted to answer a question just because you feel you have not answered enough questions to pass. The examiners often delete questions from the final analysis for various reasons and so it is often possible to score a higher percentage than you think you have because questions that you did not answer have been removed in this way. The sort of questions which can be removed include those which nobody gets right because they are too hard or which everybody gets right because they are too easy. Such questions can be deemed

# Examination technique and preparation

nondiscriminating and may be taken from the analysis.

It is important not to be put off by questions which seem slightly ambiguous. These questions occur again and again and it is usually quite possible to work out exactly what is being asked if you take the questions at face value. An example would be:

The following is characteristic of heart failure
   (a) a low jugular venous pressure
   Answer: False

It could rightly be argued that many patients with heart failure are on diuretics and are sometimes overdiuresed, so lowering the jugular venous pressure. However, the question asks quite specifically whether the low jugular pressure is *characteristic* of heart failure, not whether it may occur under certain undefined conditions. Clearly it is a raised jugular venous pressure that is truly characteristic of heart failure and not a low jugular venous pressure and so the correct answer is false. It is important to remember that you do not have a chance to communicate subtle thoughts to the examiner and so you must answer using the reply which is most likely to be right.

When doing the examination or practice questions, do not worry if you don't know an answer; the worry will certainly not help and will probably worsen your performance. One aspect of the examination which often puts candidates off is the habit the examiners have of putting in some almost impossible questions. As I have mentioned above, these will be equally hard for everyone, so if you don't know the answers just leave them out, put them out of your mind and move on to answer the next question. Under no circumstances worry about these questions while you are doing the rest of the paper. The structure of individual questions sometimes follows a certain pattern with three of the answer stems being reasonably challenging, but manageable, one being very easy and one being almost impossible. This is common and nobody else will find the difficult stems easy. Just stay calm, answer only the questions that you

Examination technique and preparation

are confident about and move on to the next question. Try to treat each question with a fresh mind uncluttered by the accumulated worries of previously unanswered questions.

**How to start**
In planning your specific preparation, bear in mind that the most valid demonstrations of what the examination is really like are the past papers published by the Royal Colleges. For this reason I suggest the following strategy. Start right away with the published past papers. Record your scores and think carefully about the questions that you got wrong. Think closely about the design of the questions and the level of certainty you would need to score well. When you have done these questions, put them aside, recording your scores and then go through as many other multiple choice questions as you can. Nowadays there are more books available than most people have time to go through. Try to select those books which have most to offer and seem well written. In addition, do not waste time on a book which seems unreliable, out of date or which you feel has given the wrong answer to a question. In particular, select books which give thoughtful comments on the answers as this will save you the considerable time it would take to look up the topic in a textbook. The examination costs a significant amount of money to take, so if you think a book might help you pass then buy it. Even if it only helps you gain an extra mark, if that is the difference between passing and failing then the book will have paid for itself in saved re-examination fees.

About 10 days to a week before the examination it is worth repeating the Royal College past papers to remind yourself of the format and style of the real questions. It is usually encouraging to compare your scores at this time to those when you first attempted the same papers. Even taking into account that you will have seen the papers before, it will probably demonstrate to you how much better your technique for negatively marked MCQs is.

## Organizing yourself – practical points

Most preparation for the examination can be done at home. Any general preparation that you have time to do, before embarking on the main thrust of your MCQ attempts is probably best done from the comfort of an armchair or comfortable desk. Suitable references are the standard textbooks of medicine, such as the *Oxford Textbook of Medicine* or recent reviews from the major medical journals. As I have outlined above, this sort of revision is very much a luxury, to be done only if you have ample time. Assuming that this is the case, read up on the major medical topics such as strokes, myocardial infarction, HIV infection and so on. In addition to this it is probably worth while making a few brief notes to remind yourself later on about slightly tedious topics such as the classification of the hyperlipidaemias. In making any such notes, it is well worth considering the best format for these notes. When you are marking the answers to your practice questions, you will often want to rapidly remind yourself about a topic. A good method for note taking is to use small alphabetically indexed filing cards. These have the advantage of rapid access and of the discipline of limiting your note taking to the key points. Large folders of lengthy notes are seldom of much value for rapid revision and it is usually a tedious process finding exactly where the answer to your query is. Obviously, a computer with an easily accessed database or indexed word processing package could be used instead, but this probably imposes an added level of complexity to the whole process without yielding notably better results. An advantage of the index cards is that nearer to the examination you can carry around a few cards with particularly difficult to remember topics on. These cards can be clamped with an elastic band or bulldog clip and pulled out of your pocket every so often for a quick revision session, even if it is only a several second glance. Even if you opt not to do any general preparation, it is still worth keeping a few cards around for note taking as inevitably

# Examination technique and preparation

there will be topics that you will want to look up while you are doing questions.

When you get down to doing practice questions, don't rush them at first. Think carefully about each stem of each question and then decide whether you can reasonably answer the question or whether it would be wiser to leave the question unanswered. When you look at the answers, try to have in mind the degree of doubt or certainty that you had when answering as this will help you to calibrate yourself and get a feel for how to answer future questions. Even if you know the topic reasonably well, have a glance at the answer comments as they are designed to provide a quick revision of key topics or a quick clarification of common points of confusion. This may seem slow at first, but it is a positive approach and you will inevitably improve using this method. In addition, you will soon find that you are both quicker and more thorough than you were initially.

It is very much a personal preference how many questions you do at a time before looking at the answers. Some people prefer to look at the answers to each question immediately after answering it. This certainly provides immediate feedback, but it can be quite tiresome flicking backwards and forwards between the questions and the answers. Probably the best approach is to do one page of questions or a set of 5–10 questions at a time, because if you are doing larger numbers of questions all at once it is easy to forget the issues the earlier questions raised for you by the time you are looking at the answers. Once again, do not waste time on practice question books that seem out of date, unreliable, or that do not give adequate explanations of the answers.

One approach that some people do find helpful is to carry a book around with them during the day or on call and just dip into it from time to time like a quiz book. It can even be profitable to do this with one or more fellow candidates in the way that a group of people might do a crossword together in the mess. Although it sounds tedious, this is often a relatively painless way of getting through more material and can be a good way of pooling the specialist knowledge which each person has built up.

## Sitting the examination

Although taking the examination can seem very daunting, in reality it is straightforward and a few sensible steps can make it less stressful. Make sure that you know exactly where the examination is taking place and how to get there well in advance. This eliminates any last minute anxiety associated with trying to find the examination location. Although writing materials may be available, you will feel more comfortable if you already have your own pens, pencils, rubbers and pencil sharpeners in your pockets. When you take your seat, spend a few moments collecting your thoughts and making sure that you are calm and level headed before you start the paper. The examination is computer marked and as the format for this can change, it is essential that you read the written instructions and listen to any verbal instructions that you are given.

Think carefully about each question, decide on your answer and then move on to the next question. Don't keep worrying about a question you are unsure of. If you are unsure don't answer the question and move on to the next one. Similarly, divide your time up sensibly and don't waste time pondering a question that you are unsure of, simply leave it out. It is worth keeping a note of the questions that you are unsure of, as if you have spare time at the end of the examination then review these questions first. However, even then do not be tempted to answer them if you are not confident that you are right. As well as knowledge, the outcome of the examination will depend on how well you can judge when to answer and when not to answer a question. By using the approach that I have outlined in this chapter, you should have a good feel for this by the time of the examination, so think carefully how you would answer the

## Examination technique and preparation

question if you were doing it for practice at home.

Lastly, it is important to stay calm and not be frightened by the examination. Most people pass it eventually and your performance is likely to be worse if you are very anxious. Be confident and calm and you will perform at your best.

# Questions

# Cardiology

**1 In the normal cardiac cycle**
   (a) the third heart sound represents atrial systole
   (b) the jugular venous pulse $x$ descent represents opening of the tricuspid valve
   (c) the heart rate is slower in expiration during sinus arrhythmia
   (d) a dicrotic notch in the carotid pulse represents aortic valve closure
   (e) the jugular venous pulse falls on expiration

**2 The following are true of the QTc interval on the electrocardiograph**
   (a) prolongation can be associated with a gene encoding a potassium channel
   (b) hypocalcaemia can prolong the QTc interval
   (c) lignocaine can prolong the QTc interval
   (d) Romano–Ward syndrome can prolong the QTc interval
   (e) quinidine can prolong the Qtc interval

**3 On auscultation of the second heart sound**
   (a) aortic stenosis can cause a reversed split
   (b) mitral regurgitation can cause a wide split
   (c) a wide split occurs in right bundle branch block
   (d) on inspiration, the pulmonary valve closes first
   (e) a patent ductus arteriosus causes a reversed split

**4 Potassium causes the following changes on the ECG (electrocardiogram)**
   (a) peaked T waves in hyperkalaemia

## Questions • Cardiology

(b) a long P–R interval in hypokalaemia
(c) loss of U waves in hypokalaemia
(d) loss of P waves in hyperkalaemia
(e) a narrow QRS complex in hyperkalaemia

### 5 In constrictive pericarditis
(a) the jugular venous pressure (JVP) rises on inspiration
(b) an early diastolic sound is characteristic
(c) pulsus paradoxus is by definition present
(d) the *y* descent in the JVP is lost
(e) the best management is urgent pericardial needle aspiration

### 6 The following are causes of cyanosis in the neonate
(a) a severe Ebstein's anomaly with an atrial septal defect (ASD)
(b) patent ductus arteriosus
(c) a primum atrial septal defect
(d) a ventricular septal defect involving the infundibulum
(e) aortic stenosis with a ventricular septal defect (VSD)

### 7 In the cardiac action potential
(a) the resting intracellular membrane potential is negative with respect to the extracellular potential
(b) it is principally sodium ions that determine the resting membrane potential
(c) initial depolarization occurs when sodium conductance increases
(d) calcium plays a role in the plateau phase of the cardiac action potential
(e) lignocaine affects sodium conductance during depolarization.

### 8 The following are true of aspirin
(a) it reduces mortality, but not reinfarction after a first

myocardial infarction
(b) it is absolutely contra-indicated in chronic renal failure
(c) peptic ulcer prophylaxis is mandatory if given with thrombolytic agents
(d) it inhibits platelet aggregation
(e) it selectively blocks endothelial prostacyclin I production

## 9 The following are features of mitral stenosis

(a) a loud second heart sound
(b) haemoptysis
(c) prophylactic digoxin should be started
(d) a raised pulmonary artery wedge pressure
(e) as severity increases the interval between the second heart sound and opening snap diminishes

## 10 Congestive heart failure

(a) is always caused by ischaemic heart disease
(b) is associated with low left ventricular end diastolic pressures
(c) is characterized by reduced sodium excretion in the absence of diuretics
(d) is associated with abnormally low peripheral resistance
(e) occurs as a result of *Trypanosoma cruzi* infection

## 11 The following are true of coronary artery disease

(a) at a serum cholesterol of 4.5 mmol the risk is negligible
(b) HDL (high density lipoprotein) – cholesterol may reduce the risk
(c) left anterior descending artery thrombosis causes inferior myocardial infarction
(d) second degree heart block in inferior myocardial infarction usually recovers
(e) beta blockers reduce mortality in myocardial infarction

**Questions** • Cardiology

## 12 In non-Q wave myocardial infarction
(a) there is a higher risk of reinfarction than in Q wave infarction
(b) the basic pathology is a stenosis of a coronary artery
(c) diltiazem is of benefit
(d) early investigation is unrewarding
(e) early mortality is low

## 13 The following are associated with thoracic aortic dissection
(a) syphilis
(b) homocystinuria
(c) hypertension
(d) coarctation of the aorta
(e) ankylosing spondylitis

## 14 The following suggest a supra-ventricular tachycardia rather than a ventricular tachycardia
(a) cannon waves in the jugular venous pulse
(b) a third heart sound
(c) fusion beats on the electrocardiograph
(d) a broad QRS complex on the electrocardiograph
(e) a response to adenosine

## 15 Aortic regurgitation occurs in
(a) the seronegative spondyloarthropathies
(b) syphilis
(c) relapsing polychondritis
(d) osteogenesis imperfecta
(e) infective endocarditis

## 16 The following are causes of right axis deviation on the electrocardiograph
(a) dextrocardia
(b) left posterior hemiblock
(c) hypokalaemia

(d) a primum atrial septal defect
(e) pulmonary emboli

**17** A slow pulse rate is characteristic in the following
(a) first degree heart block
(b) digoxin toxicity
(c) primary hypothyroidism
(d) raised intracranial pressure
(e) Gaucher's disease

**18** In the Wolff–Parkinson–White syndrome
(a) atrial fibrillation can be dangerous
(b) a class 4 antiarrhythmic is the drug of choice
(c) with a left sided bundle of Kent the QRS complex is usually positive in lead V1
(d) delta waves occur
(e) paroxysmal atrial fibrillation is the commonest dysrhythmia

**19** The following are true of catecholamines
(a) dopamine is not a positive inotrope
(b) dobutamine acts on beta-1 receptors as an agonist
(c) isoprenaline acts only on alpha adrenergic receptors
(d) salbutamol is both a beta-2 agonist and a beta-1 blocker
(e) adrenaline is only an agonist on beta-1 receptors

**20** The following are recognized features of aortic stenosis
(a) sudden death
(b) atrioventricular block
(c) an association with bicuspid valves
(d) impaired myocardial oxygen delivery
(e) a peak systolic aortic valve gradient of 100 mmHg signifies severe disease

# Endocrinology

## 1 The following are true of steroid metabolism
(a) cholesterol is a precursor of most hormonal steroids
(b) progesterone is a precursor of cortisol
(c) testosterone can be converted to oestrogens
(d) finasteride inhibits the conversion of testosterone to dihydrotestosterone by 5-alpha-reductase
(e) 5-alpha-reductase deficiency causes congenital adrenal hyperplasia with over-virilization of female babies

## 2 The following are causes of hypoglycaemia
(a) acute liver failure
(b) insulinoma
(c) sulphonylureas
(d) Addison's disease
(e) Type I (von Gierke) glycogen storage disease

## 3 The following are true of growth hormone
(a) levels are higher at night than during the day
(b) a glucose tolerance test normally causes a fall in growth hormone
(c) excess can cause carpal tunnel syndrome
(d) glucose tolerance is normal in acromegaly
(e) growth hormone acts in part through a hepatic product somatomedin C (insulin-like growth factor 1)

## 4 In hyperthyroidism the following statements are true
(a) the commonest cause is Graves disease
(b) a low TSH (thyroid stimulating hormone) and a normal thyroxine together exclude the diagnosis
(c) raised total thyroxine levels in a pregnant woman are diagnostic
(d) the diagnosis is excluded if administration of TSH

releasing hormone (TRH) causes a rise in TSH levels
(e) carbimazole inhibits thyroid hormone synthesis

## 5 The following are causes of a proximal myopathy
(a) vitamin D deficiency
(b) Cushing's syndrome
(c) polymyositis
(d) Duchenne muscular dystrophy
(e) growth hormone excess

## 6 The following are true of polycystic ovary syndrome
(a) infertility is common
(b) cysts are usually too small to be visible on ultrasound scanning
(c) testosterone levels are high
(d) the ratio of luteinising hormone to follicle stimulating hormone is abnormal
(e) there is usually a family history of polycystic kidney disease

## 7 The following are associated with osteoporosis
(a) Cushing's syndrome
(b) heparin
(c) hypogonadism
(d) warfarin
(e) rheumatoid arthritis

## 8 The following are causes of polyuria
(a) polydipsia
(b) hypercalcaemia
(c) lithium toxicity
(d) chlorpropamide
(e) acute tubular necrosis

**Questions** • Endocrinology

9 **The following are associated with galactorrhoea**
   (a) infertility
   (b) phenothiazines
   (c) frusemide
   (d) prolactinoma
   (e) acromegaly

10 **The following are true of testicular feminization syndrome**
   (a) there are always two X chromosomes
   (b) testosterone levels are always low
   (c) the phenotype is female
   (d) female secondary sexual characteristics occur with a male genotype
   (e) infertility is common

11 **The following general statements are true of insulin dependent diabetes mellitus**
   (a) good control reduces the onset of retinopathy in insulin dependent diabetes
   (b) good control slows the progression of nephropathy in insulin dependent diabetes
   (c) good control reduces the onset of neuropathy in insulin dependent diabetes
   (d) angiotensin converting enzyme inhibition slows the deterioration of diabetic nephropathy
   (e) it is an independent risk factor for ischaemic heart disease

12 **In the management of noninsulin dependent diabetes mellitus**
   (a) biguanides can cause hypoglycaemia
   (b) dietary measures are only necessary when no drug treatment is planned
   (c) sulphonylureas stimulate insulin secretion
   (d) correction of obesity can reduce the need for therapy
   (e) alpha-glucosidase inhibition may be useful

## Endocrinology • Questions

**13** The following statements are true of calcium and phosphate metabolism
(a) parathyroid hormone stimulates renal phosphate excretion
(b) hypercalcaemia stimulates parathyroid hormone secretion
(c) serum calcium is high in secondary hyperparathyroidism
(d) subperiosteal bone resorption can occur in hyperparathyroidism
(e) chronic renal failure can cause primary hyperparathyroidism

**14** The following statements relating to corticosteroids are true
(a) cortisol levels fall during the night
(b) a pituitary adenoma can cause Cushing's disease
(c) a fall in blood glucose stimulates a rise in cortisol level
(d) dexamethasone suppresses cortisol secretion
(e) excess corticosteroid can cause sodium retention by the kidney

**15** In considering post menopausal hormone replacement therapy, the following statements are true
(a) unopposed oestrogen therapy reduces the risk of coronary artery disease
(b) progestogen deficiency is the key cause of osteoporosis
(c) total cholesterol is reduced by unopposed oestrogen therapy
(d) the risk of bone fracture is reduced by hormone replacement therapy
(e) unopposed oestrogen reduces the risk of endometrial cancer

**16** The following are true of phaeochromocytomas
(a) hypertension is a recognized feature
(b) raised urinary 5-hydroxyindoleacetic acid levels occur

## Questions • Endocrinology

    (c) there is an association with myocarditis
    (d) beta blockers must be given before alpha blockers
    (e) neurofibromatosis

**17 The following may complicate diabetes mellitus**
    (a) postural hypotension
    (b) urinary retention
    (c) shortening of the QT interval on the electrocardiograph
    (d) impaired gastric emptying
    (e) prostatic cancer

**18 The following statements about thyroid cancer are true**
    (a) hyperthyroidism is usual
    (b) elevated calcitonin levels may occur with medullary carcinoma
    (c) anaplastic tumours typically occur in the young
    (d) papillary tumours have the worst prognosis
    (e) follicular tumours are the commonest

**19 The following changes normally occur in pregnancy**
    (a) an increase in the size of the pituitary gland
    (b) prolactin levels rise
    (c) glomerular filtration rate increases and serum creatinine falls
    (d) pulse rate rises
    (e) luteinising hormone and follicular stimulating hormone levels rise

**20 The following are causes of infertility**
    (a) Klinefelter's syndrome
    (b) Turner's syndrome
    (c) polycystic ovary syndrome
    (d) hyperprolactinaemia
    (e) chronic renal failure

# Gastroenterology

**1 The following statements are true of *Helicobacter pylori***
   (a) eradication reduces duodenal ulcer recurrence
   (b) its presence increases the risk of gastric adenocarcinoma
   (c) it is present in the majority of patients with duodenal ulcers
   (d) it is associated with gastric mucosa associated lymphoid tissue (MALT) lymphoma
   (e) it is a cause of antral gastritis

**2 The following are consistent with malabsorption**
   (a) low serum calcium
   (b) low serum albumin
   (c) steatorrhoea
   (d) a raised prothrombin time
   (e) neuropathy

**3 The following statements are true**
   (a) gastrin is produced by G cells in the gastric antrum
   (b) secretin stimulates pancreatic bicarbonate secretion
   (c) glucagon is mainly produced by the liver
   (d) atropine reduces the gastric acid production in response to gastrin
   (e) excess vasoactive intestinal peptide can cause secretory diarrhoea

**4 The following statements are true of acute pancreatitis**
   (a) the second most important cause in western Europe is alcohol
   (b) azathioprine is a recognized cause
   (c) scorpion venom is a recognized cause
   (d) urgent endoscopic removal of impacted gallstones improves mortality

## Questions • Gastroenterology

(e) a retinopathy with flame shaped haemorrhages is associated

### 5 In hepatitis C virus infection
(a) the main route of transmission is parenteral
(b) the virus is a single stranded RNA virus
(c) enzyme linked immunosorbent assay (ELISA) is now a highly sensitive screening test
(d) the most sensitive diagnostic test is a cDNA-PCR (polymerase chain reaction) based assay
(e) cirrhosis is common even with normal serum ALT (alanine aminotransferase) levels

### 6 In peptic ulcer disease
(a) smoking promotes ulcer recurrence
(b) ulcer complications of nonsteroidal anti-inflammatory drugs (NSAIDs) are lower in the elderly
(c) the risk association with ibuprofen is less than with piroxicam
(d) there is excess acid production in about one third of duodenal ulcer patients
(e) Zollinger–Ellison syndrome is always associated with *Helicobacter pylori* infection

### 7 The following are associated with diarrhoea
(a) Zollinger–Ellison syndrome
(b) hypogammaglobulinaemia
(c) an early peak on a lactulose breath test
(d) chronic pancreatitis
(e) Whipple's disease

### 8 In irritable bowel syndrome
(a) the majority of patients are symptom free by 5 years
(b) lactose intolerance may coexist
(c) the erythrocyte sedimentation rate is usually raised

(d) an association with noncardiac chest pain occurs
(e) the prevalence of psychiatric disorders may be increased

## 9 The following are true of chronic liver disease
(a) in chronic persistent hepatitis the prognosis is good
(b) in chronic active hepatitis autoimmune disease is the main cause
(c) ursodeoxycholic acid is of benefit in primary biliary cirrhosis
(d) alcohol related chronic active hepatitis invariably progresses to cirrhosis without abstinence
(e) beta blockers must be avoided

## 10 In a patient with a large liver, jaundice and ascites the following should be considered
(a) micronodular cirrhosis associated with alcohol
(b) constrictive pericarditis
(c) hepatoma
(d) Budd–Chiari syndrome
(e) autoimmune chronic active hepatitis

## 11 The following features of Crohn's disease may help distinguish it from ulcerative colitis.
(a) fever
(b) a lymphocytic infiltrate
(c) granuloma formation
(d) arthropathy which always responds to resection of the affected bowel
(e) long-term remission in response to an elemental diet

## 12 The following associations are real
(a) small bowel strictures and nonsteroidal anti-inflammatory use
(b) ileal ulcers and Behçet's disease
(c) cryoglobulinaemia and hepatitis C virus

(d) Whipple's disease and penicillamine use
(e) partial villous atrophy and human immunodeficiency virus

## 13 The following are true of gastrointestinal infections
(a) erythema nodosum can occur with *Yersinia enterocolitica* infection
(b) reactive arthritis can follow campylobacter infection
(c) cryptosporidium must always be treated
(d) schistosomiasis can cause portal hypertension
(e) *Giardia lamblia* can cause prolonged malabsorption

## 14 In the carcinoid syndrome
(a) hepatic metastasis is only present in a minority of patients
(b) pulmonary valve disease is a recognized association
(c) octreotide is of benefit
(d) diarrhoea can occur
(e) a nuclear octreotide scan can image the disease

## 15 Sclerosing cholangitis is associated with the following
(a) ulcerative colitis in the majority of patients
(b) the majority of patients are women
(c) antimitochondrial antibodies are positive
(d) ursodeoxycholic acid improves prognosis
(e) liver biopsy is the best way of making the diagnosis

## 16 The following are causes of dysphagia
(a) achalasia
(b) systemic sclerosis
(c) diabetes mellitus
(d) Chagas' disease
(e) cystic fibrosis

Gastroenterology • **Questions**

**17 In the presence of oesophageal acid reflux the following may occur**
(a) recurrent pulmonary infection
(b) a respiratory alkalosis
(c) columnar epithelialization of the lower oesophagus
(d) exacerbation of asthma
(e) diffuse alveolar haemorrhage

**18 In the presence of adult pyloric stenosis secondary to peptic ulceration the following may occur**
(a) alkalosis
(b) hypokalaemia
(c) aspiration pneumonia
(d) inappropriately acid urine
(e) reduced glomerular filtration rate

**19 In acute liver failure**
(a) hypoglycaemia is well recognized
(b) cerebral oedema is the leading cause of death in advanced acute liver failure
(c) barbiturates may be of benefit when cerebral oedema occurs
(d) lactulose is given in the presence of encephalopathy
(e) liver transplantation is contra-indicated in the presence of encephalopathy

**20 The following are associated with chronic liver disease**
(a) cystic fibrosis
(b) hepatitis C virus
(c) alkaptonuria
(d) porphyria cutanea tarda
(e) Bartter's syndrome

# Haematology

1 **The following are associated with a megaloblastic anaemia**
   (a) coeliac disease
   (b) pernicious anaemia
   (c) phenytoin
   (d) pregnancy
   (e) alcohol abuse

2 **The following are associated with thrombocytopaenia**
   (a) heparin
   (b) haemolytic uraemic syndrome
   (c) antiphospholipid antibodies
   (d) von Willebrand's disease
   (e) idiopathic membranous nephropathy

3 **The following drugs potentiate the anticoagulant effects of warfarin**
   (a) phenytoin
   (b) cimetidine
   (c) rifampicin
   (d) sulphonamides
   (e) thiopentone

4 **Sickle cell disease may result in the following**
   (a) hypoxia
   (b) dactylitis
   (c) osteomyelitis
   (d) hyposplenism
   (e) nephropathy

5 **A large liver and spleen are usually found in:**
   (a) beta-thalassaemia major
   (b) schistosomiasis

(c) leishmaniasis
(d) aplastic anaemia
(e) beta-thalassaemia trait

6 **The following statements are true**
(a) in paroxysmal nocturnal haemoglobinuria erythrocytes are damaged by complement
(b) mycoplasma infection is often associated with cryoglobulins
(c) in vitamin $B_{12}$ deficiency red cell transketolase activity is reduced
(d) vitamin $B_{12}$ levels can be high in chronic granulocytic leukaemia
(e) the Philadelphia chromosome is characteristic of chronic lymphatic leukaemia

7 **The following statements about haemoglobin are true**
(a) it exists normally as a tetramer of four haem containing rings
(b) the sigmoid oxygen dissociation curve results from co-operativity of oxygen binding between the four chains
(c) 2,3-diphosphoglycerate increases the oxygen affinity
(d) mutations in the DNA upstream of the coding sequence can cause thalassaemia
(e) normally there are four functioning alpha-haemoglobin genes in adults

8 **In acute myeloid leukaemia the following are typically found**
(a) a peak incidence in childhood
(b) rearrangements of the T cell receptor genes
(c) thrombocytopaenia
(d) a better prognosis than acute lymphatic leukaemia
(e) nephrotic syndrome

## Questions • Haematology

**9 In chronic granulocytic leukaemia the following are true**
   (a) transformation to acute leukaemia occurs in most patients
   (b) massive hepatosplenomegaly may occur
   (c) chemotherapy is often curative
   (d) the white blood cell count is usually low
   (e) the peak incidence is between 50 and 60 years

**10 A systemic thrombophilia may occur as a result of**
   (a) lupus anticoagulant
   (b) an inherited resistance to the effects of protein C
   (c) factor V Leiden
   (d) nephrotic syndrome
   (e) protein S deficiency

**11 In the investigation of a microcytic anaemia**
   (a) a raised ferritin can be present with iron deficiency
   (b) an alpha-thalassaemia could be responsible
   (c) total iron binding capacity is increased with iron deficiency
   (d) iron deficiency usually reflects blood loss in the UK
   (e) a sideroblastic anaemia could be responsible

**12 In glucose-6-phosphate deficiency the following drugs may be hazardous**
   (a) chloroquine
   (b) sulphonamide
   (c) nitrofurantoin
   (d) aspirin
   (e) dapsone

**13 The following statements are true of myeloma**
   (a) renal impairment can arise from the presence of light chain casts in the tubules
   (b) renal failure is a poor prognostic sign
   (c) anaemia is not a poor prognostic sign

(d) normal immunoglobulin levels may be reduced
(e) myeloma cells produce osteoclast activating factor

## 14 Hyperviscosity syndrome is associated with the following
(a) myeloma
(b) Waldenström's macroglobulinaemia
(c) a response to plasmapheresis
(d) neuropathy
(e) retinopathy

## 15 The following statements concerning blood clotting are true
(a) factor VII is vitamin K dependent
(b) haemophilia prolongs the activated partial thromboplastin time
(c) von Willebrand's disease prolongs the bleeding time
(d) plasmin promotes the formation of fibrin from fibrinogen
(e) chronic renal failure prolongs bleeding time

## 16 During the development of blood cells
(a) adult B cell production occurs principally in the liver
(b) interleukin-6 is an important growth factor for myeloma
(c) many T cell precursors are destroyed in the thymus
(d) tissue macrophages can become circulating monocytes
(e) granulocyte-macrophage colony stimulating factor (GM-CSF) promotes monocyte production

## 17 A low haemoglobin can occur as a result of
(a) gastrointestinal loss in rheumatoid arthritis
(b) erythropoetin deficiency in focal segmental glomerulosclerosis
(c) auto-immune haemolysis with chronic lymphocytic leukaemia
(d) bleeding in Ehlers–Danlos syndrome
(e) aplastic anaemia with phenylbutazone therapy

## Questions • Haematology/Infection

**18 The following statements concerning lymphomas are true**
(a) coeliac disease is a risk factor for small bowel lymphoma
(b) in Hodgkin's disease night sweats are not B symptoms
(c) mycosis fungoides has a poor prognosis
(d) Sézary syndrome has a good prognosis
(e) in non-Hodgkin's lymphomas, high grade disease has a worse prognosis than low grade disease

**19 The following statements are true of promyelocytic leukaemia**
(a) tretinoin (all-trans retinoic acid) is of benefit
(b) the induction of further differentiation is of therapeutic benefit
(c) a bleeding diathesis is common
(d) the retinoic acid receptor alpha ($RAR\alpha$) gene is frequently rearranged
(e) it is a form of acute lymphoblastic leukaemia

**20 The following statements concerning blood transfusion are true**
(a) naturally occurring antibodies can exist to the A and B antigens
(b) pregnancy can sensitize a baby to the D antigen of the Rhesus system
(c) ABO incompatibility causes complement activation
(d) white cell reactions can cause pulmonary infiltrates
(e) in a crossmatch donor serum is tested with recipient cells

# Infection

**1 The following are true of tetanus**
(a) the vaccine is a live attenuated vaccine
(b) the pathogen is a Gram-positive coccus

(c) persistent tonic generalized spasm can occur
(d) dysphagia can occur
(e) benzodiazepines and metronidazole are of benefit

## 2 The following are true of leprosy

(a) with lepromatous leprosy, spontaneous healing and resolution are usual
(b) tuberculoid leprosy is usually generalized
(c) in tuberculoid leprosy there may be areas of anaesthesia with thickening of peripheral nerves
(d) in tuberculoid leprosy, T helper 1 (TH1) type cells producing interleukin-2 and interferon gamma predominate
(e) BCG vaccination offers some protection against leprosy

## 3 In Lyme disease, the following are true

(a) the causative organism is a spirochaete
(b) ixodid ticks carry the organism
(c) an intermittent inflammatory arthritis can occur
(d) a migrating erythematous rash can occur
(e) a facial palsy can occur

## 4 In deciding on malaria prophylaxis and treatment the following are true

(a) chloroquine resistance is common in sub-Saharan Africa
(b) mefloquine resistance does not yet exist
(c) halofantrine can lengthen the QT interval
(d) the combination of pyrimethamine and dapsone may result in agranulocytosis
(e) in pregnancy chloroquine and proguanil have a safe record for prophylaxis

## 5 The following are true of toxacara infection

(a) the causative organism is a spirochaete
(b) eosinophilia can occur
(c) diethylcarbamazine can be useful in treatment

## Questions • Infection

   (d) retinal granulomas can occur in children
   (e) splenomegaly is not a feature

6 **In leishmaniasis the following are true**
   (a) the vector is the tetse fly
   (b) the leishmania test is negative in cutaneous leishmaniasis
   (c) raised immunoglobulin levels occur in visceral leishmaniasis
   (d) kala azar complicating HIV infection in Mediterranean countries is well recognized
   (e) amphotericin and pentavalent antimonial drugs are of benefit

7 **The following are recognized in HIV infection**
   (a) cryptococcal infection
   (b) cryptosporidial infection
   (c) *Mycobacterium kansasii* infection
   (d) cytomegalovirus retinopathy
   (e) dementia

8 **The following may result from schistosomiasis infection**
   (a) hepatosplenomegaly with portal hypertension
   (b) cor pulmonale
   (c) haematuria
   (d) hepatic granuloma formation
   (e) itch

9 **The following are true of influenza virus infection**
   (a) prominent myalgia is a feature
   (b) the virus is an RNA virus
   (c) changes in surface haemagglutinin and neuraminidase cause antigenic shift
   (d) the vaccine is contra-indicated in pregnancy
   (e) amantadine is active against influenza A

## 10 The following may cause jaundice
  (a) Epstein–Barr virus
  (b) malaria
  (c) cytomegalovirus infection
  (d) measles
  (e) varicella zoster infection

## 11 *Chlamydia trachomatis* can cause the following illnesses
  (a) sexually transmitted urethritis
  (b) psittacosis
  (c) lymphogranuloma venereum
  (d) blindness
  (e) retinopathy

## 12 The following are recognized complications of falciparum malaria
  (a) acute renal failure
  (b) hypoglycaemia
  (c) anaemia
  (d) coma
  (e) Gram-negative septicaemia

## 13 In *Salmonella typhi* infections the following are true
  (a) the organisms are Gram-positive
  (b) rose spots can occur
  (c) blood culture is of no diagnostic use
  (d) abdominal pain is common
  (e) abscess formation can occur

## 14 The following conditions can predispose to *Candida albicans* infection
  (a) broad spectrum antibiotic therapy
  (b) diabetes
  (c) steroid therapy
  (d) pregnancy
  (e) human immunodeficiency virus infection

## Questions • Infection

### 15 The following are true of amoebic disease
(a) diarrhoea with blood and mucus can occur
(b) diarrhoea can recur for years
(c) an amoebic liver abscess can occur years after the initial infection
(d) metronidazole is of no benefit
(e) serological tests are of no benefit

### 16 The following associations are real
(a) *Ascaris lumbricoides* (round worm) infection and biliary or bowel obstruction
(b) *Enterobius vermicularis* (threadworm) infection and pruritus ani
(c) *Necator americanus* (hookworm) infection and iron deficiency anaemia
(d) *Strongyloides stercoralis* infection and a recurrent itchy rash
(e) *Trichuris trichuria* (whipworm) infection and no symptoms

### 17 The following are recognized adverse effects of antituberculous therapy
(a) isoniazid and peripheral neuropathy
(b) streptomycin and impaired hearing
(c) pyrazinamide and optic neuritis
(d) ethambutol and reduced activity of the oral contraceptive pill
(e) rifampicin and liver damage

### 18 In bacterial infection the following statements are true
(a) Group A streptococci can cause rheumatic fever
(b) Group A streptococci can cause necrotising fasciitis
(c) staphylococcal food poisoning results from the presence of a toxin in the food
(d) Group B streptococci are the usual cause of post streptococcal glomerulonephritis
(e) diphtheria is a Gram-negative organism

## Infection/Nephrology • Questions

**19 The following are true of hydatid disease**
(a) the causative organism is *Taenia solium*
(b) most cysts form in the brain
(c) the disease is a zoonosis which can be transmitted by dogs
(d) cysts can become calcified
(e) eosinophilia is not a feature

**20 In a patient with advanced HIV infection the following may be true**
(a) diarrhoea can result from autonomic neuropathy
(b) prophylaxis against *Pneumocystis carinii* is of benefit
(c) CD4+ T cell counts are raised in peripheral blood
(d) the virus is an RNA virus
(e) gancyclovir used for cytomegalovirus infection may cause bone marrow suppression

# Nephrology

**1 The kidney is usually a net excreter of the following**
(a) phosphate
(b) sodium
(c) urea
(d) creatinine
(e) water

**2 The following are excreted by the kidney**
(a) cyclosporin
(b) fluconazole
(c) nitrofurantoin
(d) nifedipine
(e) hydrallazine

**Questions** • Nephrology

3 **The following or their metabolites accumulate in renal failure.**
   (a) dopamine
   (b) minoxidil
   (c) metoprolol
   (d) cimetidine
   (e) allopurinol

4 **The following are nephrotoxic**
   (a) indomethacin
   (b) cyclosporin
   (c) gentamicin
   (d) diltiazem
   (e) nitrofurantoin

5 **The following are common causes of community acquired urinary tract infection**
   (a) *Escherichia coli*
   (b) *Staphylococcus aureus*
   (c) *Proteus mirabilis*
   (d) Klebsiella species
   (e) *Candida albicans*

6 **In men with renal artery stenosis the following are common**
   (a) elevated blood pressure
   (b) elevated serum creatinine
   (c) bilateral disease
   (d) the stenosis progresses but does not occlude
   (e) captopril is the drug of choice

7 **In membranous nephropathy in adults**
   (a) nephrotic syndrome is uncommon
   (b) most patients progress to end stage renal disease
   (c) an underlying malignancy is found in most cases

(d) spontaneous remission is common
(e) frank haematuria is common

## 8 The following can decrease renal blood flow
(a) adrenaline
(b) low dose dopamine
(c) indomethacin
(d) captopril
(e) trimethoprim

## 9 In IgA nephropathy
(a) the prognosis is excellent with treatment
(b) frank haematuria is common
(c) children can be affected
(d) hypertension is common
(e) nephrotic syndrome is usual

## 10 In minimal change disease
(a) electron microscopy is normal
(b) immunofluorescence is positive for IgG
(c) progressive renal failure is common
(d) treatment is not usually required
(e) nephrotic syndrome is unusual

## 11 In focal segmental glomerular sclerosis
(a) the outlook is excellent for renal function
(b) nephrotic syndrome is common
(c) immunofluorescence is usually positive on a renal biopsy
(d) patients are usually elderly
(e) recurrence in transplants is uncommon

## 12 In diabetic nephropathy
(a) retinopathy is unusual
(b) haematuria is the first sign
(c) nephrotic syndrome is usual

**Questions** • Nephrology

(d) transplantation is contra-indicated because of infection.

(e) hypertension is uncommon

**13 In adults with hypertension**

(a) renal damage is seldom seen

(b) haematuria is common

(c) proteinuria is usually heavy if present

(d) most cases have an underlying cause

(e) treatment should not be started unless the diastolic blood pressure is raised

**14 The following are well recognized causes of renal diseases**

(a) penicillamine

(b) hydrallazine

(c) gold

(d) acyclovir

(e) amphotericin

**15 In the nephrotic syndrome**

(a) there is sodium retention

(b) there is a tendency to thrombosis

(c) immune function is normal

(d) protein restriction is recommended

(e) serum lipids are lowered

**16 In renal tubular acidosis the following are true**

(a) urine is too acid

(b) potassium is always normal

(c) serum chloride concentrations are low

(d) angiotensin converting enzyme inhibitors are helpful in most cases

(e) the plasma anion gap is increased

**17 The following are causes of nephrocalcinosis**

(a) hyperparathyroidism

(b) distal renal tubular acidosis
(c) medullary sponge kidney
(d) sarcoidosis
(e) milk alkali syndrome

## 18 In polycystic kidney disease
(a) the adult disease is recessive
(b) the juvenile disease is dominant
(c) end stage renal disease is inevitable
(d) cerebrovascular thrombosis is an association
(e) the gene for the adult disease is on chromosome 16

## 19 The following are associated with end stage renal disease
(a) erythrocytosis
(b) hyperparathyroidism
(c) increased cardiovascular mortality
(d) amyloidosis
(e) peptic ulceration

## 20 The following are true of Goodpasture's disease
(a) there are antibodies to glomerular basement membrane
(b) the condition can be fatal
(c) plasma exchange is of no benefit
(d) diffuse alveolar haemorrhage can occur
(e) most patients are women

# Neurology

## 1 The following statements are true
(a) the middle cerebral artery supplies the basal ganglia and internal capsule
(b) the basilar artery divides to form the posterior cerebral arteries

(c) noradrenaline is the key neurotransmitter in the parasympathetic system
(d) the spinal cord ends at L5
(e) the cavernous sinus drains into the internal jugular vein via the petrosal sinuses

## 2 Vitamin $B_{12}$ deficiency may cause the following
(a) optic atrophy
(b) megaloblastic anaemia
(c) paraesthesia
(d) distal sensory loss
(e) areflexia

## 3 The following are true of ischaemic stroke
(a) aspirin reduces the risk among patients with normal valves and atrial fibrillation
(b) warfarin reduces the risk among patients with normal valves and atrial fibrillation
(c) surgery is the preferred therapy in patients with symptomatic severe carotid stenosis
(d) in healthy middle aged men aspirin reduces death from strokes.
(e) systolic hypertension is not an independent risk factor for stroke

## 4 The following statements are true of prion related disease
(a) transmissible prions consist of an abnormal form of a normal cellular protein
(b) Creutzfeldt–Jakob disease can be inherited, transmissible or sporadic
(c) amyloid plaques can be deposited in human prion disease
(d) Creutzfeldt–Jakob disease can cause myoclonus and fits
(e) Kuru is associated with tribal cannibalism

## Neurology • Questions

**5** The following are associated with an increased risk of stroke
   (a) diabetes mellitus
   (b) systolic hypertension
   (c) psoriasis
   (d) antiphospholipid syndrome
   (e) left atrial myxoma

**6** In multiple sclerosis the following are true
   (a) peripheral demyelination is usual
   (b) the concordance is higher in monozygotic than dizygotic twins
   (c) helper CD4+ T cells are found in acute lesions
   (d) the appearances on magnetic resonance imaging are not found with other diseases
   (e) visual evoked potentials are often delayed

**7** The following are causes of palpably thickened peripheral nerves
   (a) amyloidosis
   (b) folate deficiency
   (c) leprosy
   (d) hypothyroidism
   (e) alcohol

**8** The dorsal columns of the spinal cord are
   (a) supplied with blood by the posterior spinal arteries
   (b) play the major role in temperature sensation
   (c) can be affected by vitamin $B_{12}$ deficiency
   (d) supply sensation to the ipsilateral body
   (e) are affected in Friedreich's ataxia

**9** A mononeuritis multiplex can occur in
   (a) polyarteritis nodosa
   (b) leprosy

(c) diabetes mellitus
(d) sarcoidosis
(e) amyloidosis

**10** Upgoing plantar responses and absent leg tendon reflexes are recognized features of
(a) motor neurone disease
(b) sarcoidosis
(c) myeloma
(d) vitamin $B_{12}$ deficiency
(e) Friedreich's ataxia

**11** The following diseases are associated with a predominantly sensory neuropathy
(a) diphtheria
(b) leprosy
(c) Charcot–Marie–Tooth disease
(d) acute intermittent porphyria
(e) Guillain–Barré syndrome

**12** The following may be present in myasthaenia gravis
(a) thymoma
(b) antibodies to the acetylcholine receptor
(c) sensory neuropathy
(d) a response to edrophonium bromide
(e) diplopia

**13** The following statements are true of Parkinson's disease
(a) Lewy bodies occur in the substantia nigra
(b) bladder and bowel function is not affected
(c) the tremor worsens on activity
(d) an excess of dopamine is the central problem
(e) intellectual function is unaffected

## Neurology • Questions

**14** Considering the pharmacology of 5-hydroxytryptamine (5HT or serotonin)
   (a) sumatriptan is an agonist at 5-HT1 receptors
   (b) tricyclic antidepressants inhibit 5-HT reuptake at synapses
   (c) ondansetron is an antagonist of 5-HT
   (d) sumatriptan causes vasodilation
   (e) fluoxetine inhibits 5-HT reuptake at synapses

**15** The following may occur in vitamin $B_1$ deficiency
   (a) impaired myocardial function
   (b) reduced red blood cell transketolase activity
   (c) irreversible neurological damage
   (d) nystagmus
   (e) symmetrical polyneuropathy

**16** The following features may occur in *Borrelia burgdorferei* infection
   (a) cranial polyneuropathy
   (b) arthropathy
   (c) lymphocytic meningitis
   (d) an erythematous migratory rash
   (e) acute renal failure

**17** The following cause predominantly distal weakness on testing muscle power
   (a) Charcot–Marie–Tooth disease
   (b) Duchenne muscular dystrophy
   (c) dystrophia myotonica
   (d) Wilson's disease
   (e) Huntington's disease

**18** In the unconscious patient
   (a) the pathway of the pupillary light reflex passes through the occipital cortex
   (b) the presence of doll's eyes movements confirms brainstem damage

**Questions** • Neurology/Pharmacology

(c) the doll's eyes reflex involves the medial longitudinal fasciculus
(d) the corneal reflex afferent pathway is the trigeminal nerve
(e) cocaine use may cause large reactive pupils

**19 The following are causes of increases in cerebrospinal fluid protein content and lymphocyte count**
(a) sarcoidosis
(b) syphilis
(c) herpes simplex infection
(d) tuberculosis
(e) motor neurone disease

**20 In ischaemic stroke the following correlations are usual**
(a) a right inferior quadrantic homonymous hemianopia with a left parietal cortex lesion
(b) expressive dysphasia with a dominant temporal lobe lesion
(c) greater paralysis in the left leg than the left arm with a right anterior cerebral artery occlusion
(d) weakness affecting the right arm and leg with a left internal capsule lesion
(e) a contralateral leg and arm paralysis with a midbrain lesion

# Pharmacology

**1 When prescribing monoamine oxidase inhibitors the following are true**
(a) monoamine oxidase A preferentially acts on noradenaline and 5-hydroxytryptamine and monoamine oxidase B preferentially acts on phenylethylamine
(b) selegiline preferentially inhibits monoamine oxidase A

(c) tyramine containing foods can cause profound hypotension in the presence of monoamine oxidase inhibition
(d) in the presence of monoamine oxidase inhibition tricyclic antidepressants can cause severe hypertension
(e) pethidine can safely be used with monoamine oxidase inhibitors

## 2 The following statements concerning 5-hydroxytryptamine (5HT) are true

(a) sumatriptan is an agonist at receptors in intracranial blood vessels
(b) fluoxetine and fluvoxamine inhibit 5-hydroxytryptamine reuptake by neurones
(c) ondansetron is a 5-hydroxytryptamine agonist
(d) serotonin and 5-hydroxytryptamine are different substances
(e) sumatriptan can cause coronary vasoconstriction

## 3 Cocaine can have the following effects

(a) acute myocardial infarction
(b) overdose can cause hypertension and tachycardia
(c) pupillary constriction
(d) convulsions if taken in overdose
(e) nasal septal perforation

## 4 In the treatment of supraventricular tachycardias the following statements are true

(a) adenosine stimulates an outward potassium current in supraventricular tissue
(b) adenosine causes hyperpolarization of atrial cells
(c) aminophylline enhances the effects of adenosine
(d) bronchospasm may be exacerbated in asthmatics by adenosine
(e) verapamil is safer than adenosine for broad complex tachycardias

## Questions • Pharmacology

### 5 The following statements concerning nitric oxide are true
(a) it is synthesized from L-arginine by the vascular endothelium
(b) it has a half life of several days
(c) it is a vasoconstrictor
(d) severe infection reduces the production of nitric oxide
(e) there are no known inhibitors of nitric oxide production

### 6 In the treatment of diabetes the following are true
(a) sulphonylureas stimulate insulin secretion
(b) chlorpropamide has a longer half life than tolbutamide
(c) lactic acidosis can occur with metformin
(d) tight glycaemic control does not influence the development of complications
(e) dietary control is only necessary with oral hypoglycaemic agents

### 7 The following inhibit the aggregation of platelets
(a) aspirin
(b) thromboxane A2
(c) prostacyclin
(d) erythropoetin
(e) von Willebrand factor

### 8 In a patient with gout the following statements are true
(a) colchicine must never be given to a patient with renal failure
(b) allopurinol is safe in patients on azathioprine
(c) nonsteroidal anti-inflammatory drugs should be avoided in patients taking allopurinol
(d) low dose aspirin inhibits urate excretion
(e) thiazide diuretics are of benefit

## 9 The following are recognized complications of drugs used in cancer chemotherapy

(a) cyclophosphamide and haemorrhagic cystitis
(b) adriamycin and dilated cardiomyopathy
(c) cisplatin and nephrotoxicity
(d) vincristine and peripheral neuropathy
(e) bleomycin and pulmonary fibrosis

## 10 The following drugs have proven prophylactic value for the conditions mentioned

(a) cotrimoxazole for *Pneumocystis carinii* infection
(b) aspirin for secondary prevention of myocardial infarction
(c) ondansetron for cytotoxic drug induced vomiting
(d) thiamine for isoniazid induced peripheral neuropathy
(e) ciprofloxacin for traveller's diarrhoea

## 11 The following drugs would be sensible antihypertensives in the given clinical settings

(a) a thiazide diuretic in a diabetic
(b) an angiotensin converting enzyme inhibitor in a patient on dialysis
(c) labetalol in a pregnant woman
(d) propranolol in a patient with peripheral vascular disease
(e) nifedipine while breastfeeding

## 12 The following drug combinations are generally sensible

(a) rifampicin and the oral contraceptive pill
(b) frusemide and triamterene
(c) chlorpromazine and L-dopa
(d) adrenaline and dopamine
(e) salbutamol and atenolol

## 13 The following are correct mechanisms of action for the drugs concerned

(a) acyclovir inhibits a herpes virus thymidine kinase

## Questions • Pharmacology

(b) ampicillin inhibits protein synthesis in bacteria

(c) pyridostigmine blocks acetylcholine receptors

(d) benzodiazepines act on gamma-amino-butyric acid receptors

(e) atropine inhibits adrenergic transmission

**14** The following are complications of total parenteral nutrition

(a) air embolism

(b) elevated liver enzyme tests

(c) hyperglycaemia

(d) hypophosphataemia

(e) Type 1 hyperlipidaemia (chylomicronaemia)

**15** The following statements concerning catecholaminergic action are true

(a) salbutamol acts principally by a beta-agonist effect

(b) mefenamic acid is an alpha blocker

(c) dopamine has beta-1 agonist activity

(d) atenolol can exacerbate asthma

(e) bradycardia can result from isoprenaline

**16** The following are true of paracetamol

(a) hepatocellular necrosis can occur with an overdose

(b) *N*-acetyl-cysteine supplies glutathione

(c) the drug inhibits prostaglandin synthesis

(d) overdose can result in coma

(e) in overdose impaired clotting is of no significance

**17** The following drugs can cause hypokalaemia

(a) bumetanide

(b) prednisolone

(c) triamcinolone

(d) aminophylline

(e) salbutamol

## 18 The following are well recognized dermatological adverse reactions to the drugs listed
(a) erythema multiforme and sulphonamides
(b) photosensitivity and amiodarone
(c) toxic macular erythema and penicillins
(d) erythema nodosum and oestrogens
(e) exfoliative dermatitis and gold

## 19 The following drugs can cause hyponatraemia
(a) frusemide
(b) carbamazepine
(c) chlorpropamide
(d) fludrocortisone
(e) aminoglutethimide

## 20 The following are well recognized associations of overdose with the drugs mentioned
(a) aspirin overdose and metabolic alkalosis
(b) phenytoin overdose and cardiac dysrhythmia
(c) digoxin overdose and heart block
(d) amitriptylline overdose and interstitial nephritis
(e) azathioprine overdose and neutropaenia

# Respiratory

## 1 When testing respiratory function
(a) increased gas transfer can be measured in Goodpasture's syndrome
(b) increased gas transfer can be measured in asthma
(c) an increased KCO is typical of sarcoidosis
(d) a flow volume loop can distinguish extra and intrathoracic airway obstruction
(e) emphysema may increase residual volume

## Questions • Respiratory

**2 The following are true of adult asthma**
   (a) inhaled steroids form the core treatment
   (b) an underlying allergic cause is usual
   (c) there is an association with systemic vasculitis
   (d) bronchial hyper-responsiveness is usual
   (e) inpatient treatment often cause hyperkalaemia

**3 The following suggest active tuberculosis**
   (a) a positive Heaf test in an unvaccinated adult
   (b) apical calcification on a chest radiograph
   (c) a cough not responding to 3 months of ethambutol
   (d) noncaseating granulomas
   (e) a positive Congo red stain on transbronchial biopsy

**4 The following may point to a diagnosis of sarcoidosis**
   (a) chest X-ray changes
   (b) reduced urinary calcium excretion
   (c) reduced gas transfer on lung function
   (d) gallium scanning
   (e) thoracic computed tomography (CT scanning)

**5 Hypoxia may result from the following**
   (a) asthma
   (b) Fallot's tetralogy
   (c) polio
   (d) ankylosing spondylitis
   (e) working in the ceramics industry

**6 In lung disease related to coal mining the following are true**
   (a) damage usually relates to noxious gases underground
   (b) airflow is usually reduced
   (c) coal may be expectorated
   (d) Caplan's syndrome is caused by smoking
   (e) progressive massive fibrosis occurs eventually

## Respiratory • Questions

7 **In patients with a pleural effusion**
   (a) a protein concentration of 15g/l implies a transudate
   (b) a high lymphocyte count is consistent with tuberculosis
   (c) a low glucose concentration in the effusion is diagnostic of infection
   (d) constrictive pericarditis can be present
   (e) reference to the serum albumin may be helpful

8 **In the undiseased state the following are true**
   (a) arterial oxygen concentration does not increase significantly with excessive ventilation
   (b) carbon dioxide excretion is proportional to ventilation
   (c) the ratio of ventilation to perfusion is uniform throughout the lungs
   (d) the partial pressure of oxygen in the alveolar gas equals that in blood leaving the left ventricle
   (e) carbon dioxide can bind haemoglobin

9 **In disease related to aspergillus species the following are true**
   (a) there is always a history of asthma
   (b) aspergillus precipitins are positive in extrinsic allergic alveolitis
   (c) the eosinophil count is usually normal with an intracavity aspergilloma
   (d) bronchiectasis can occur
   (e) steroids are useful with pulmonary eosinophilia

10 **The following are associated with recurrent pulmonary infection from childhood**
   (a) cystic fibrosis
   (b) hypogammaglobulinaemia
   (c) Meigs' syndrome
   (d) Kartagener's syndrome
   (e) Barter's syndrome

**Questions** • Respiratory

## 11 The following are associated with pulmonary fibrosis
(a) Farmer's lung
(b) a ventricular septal defect
(c) scleroderma
(d) alpha-1-antitrypsin deficiency
(e) asbestos exposure

## 12 In lung cancer the following statements are generally true
(a) small cell lung cancer has a worse prognosis untreated than large cell lung cancer
(b) hypercalcaemia is most commonly associated with squamous cell carcinomas
(c) the commonest histological type is adenocarcinoma
(d) small cell lung cancer is invariably metastatic at presentation
(e) most patients will benefit from surgery

## 13 Pulmonary fibrosis in the following characteristically affects the upper zones
(a) ankylosing spondylitis
(b) sarcoidosis
(c) extrinsic allergic alveolitis
(d) asbestosis
(e) rheumatoid arthritis

## 14 The following are true of cystic fibrosis
(a) an affected parent is usual
(b) sweat sodium concentration is high
(c) oesophageal varices can occur
(d) colonization with *Pseudomonas cepacia* shortens life expectancy
(e) bowel obstruction can occur

## Respiratory • Questions

**15** The following are causes of a high broncho-alveolar lavage lymphocyte count
  (a) sarcoidosis
  (b) cryptogenic fibrosing alveolitis
  (c) streptococcal pneumonia
  (d) cytomegalovirus
  (e) extrinsic allergic alveolitis

**16** The following are associated with diffuse alveolar haemorrhage
  (a) Wegener's granulomatosis
  (b) systemic lupus erythematosus
  (c) Cushing's syndrome
  (d) idiopathic rapidly progressive glomerulonephritis
  (e) idiopathic pulmonary haemosiderosis

**17** Radiographic lung shadows and a peripheral blood eosinophilia can occur in
  (a) allergic bronchopulmonary aspergillosis
  (b) polyarteritis nodosa
  (c) diabetes mellitus
  (d) filariasis
  (e) alkaptonuria

**18** The following statements are true
  (a) psittacosis can be transmitted from birds to man
  (b) pigeon fanciers lung is caused by a hypersensitivity reaction
  (c) pulmonary artery wedge pressure is always high in adult respiratory distress syndrome
  (d) exposure to beryllium can cause granuloma formation
  (e) *Legionella pneumophila* is a Gram-positive rod

**Questions** • Respiratory/Rheumatology

### 19 The following are true of *Mycoplasma pneumoniae* infections
(a) the organism has a thick cell wall which is resistant to penicillins
(b) a meningo-encephalopathy can occur
(c) cryoglobulins are well recognized
(d) haemolysis can occur
(e) trimethoprim is effective therapy

### 20 The following are true of sleep related respiratory disorders
(a) in central sleep apnoea hypoxia does not occur
(b) obesity is a risk factor
(c) headaches are common
(d) the upper airways may collapse on expiration and open on inspiration
(e) polycythaemia may occur

# Rheumatology

### 1 In rheumatoid arthritis
(a) men are affected more than women
(b) cerebral involvement is usual
(c) a positive rheumatoid factor is diagnostic
(d) steroids are the preferred treatment
(e) symptoms are worse after exercise

### 2 In systemic lupus erythematosus
(a) joint destruction is common
(b) psychiatric disturbances are the commonest manifestation
(c) skin lesions are typically very painful
(d) there is usually proteinuria and haematuria
(e) large joints are affected first

## 3 The following are causes of muscle wasting

(a) polymyalgia rheumatica
(b) polymyositis
(c) influenza
(d) vitamin D deficiency
(e) lithium

## 4 Sjögren's syndrome

(a) is more common in women
(b) typically causes a high C reactive protein
(c) is consistent with a Schirmer's test of 20 mm in 5 min
(d) can be diagnosed by lip biopsy
(e) is associated with distal renal tubular acidosis

## 5 The following usually cause a high erythrocyte sedimentation rate (ESR)

(a) rheumatoid arthritis
(b) temporal arteritis
(c) systemic lupus erythematosus
(d) Waldenstrom's macroglobulinaemia
(e) essential mixed cryoglobulinaemia

## 6 In gout

(a) crystals are negatively birefringent under polarized light
(b) synovial fluid neutrophil count is high
(c) serum urate is high
(d) joint destruction does not occur
(e) hypertension is an association

## 7 In the assessment of back pain

(a) morning stiffness suggests depression
(b) loss of the ankle reflexes is a normal finding
(c) pain on flexion indicates facet joint disease
(d) an L4–L5 disc prolapse causes a positive sciatic nerve stretch test
(e) an L5–S1 disc prolapse causes weakness of knee extension

**Questions** • Rheumatology

### 8 Antineutrophil cytoplasmic antibodies occur in
(a) Churg–Strauss syndrome
(b) temporal arteritis
(c) systemic lupus erythematosus
(d) microscopic polyarteritis
(e) scleroderma

### 9 A rheumatoid factor
(a) is an antibody with specificity for IgM
(b) is usually present in microscopic polyarteritis
(c) is removed by dialysis
(d) may occur in the absence of joint abnormalities
(e) can occur in infective endocarditis

### 10 In a patient with psoriasis
(a) there is no treatment which alters the course of the joint disease
(b) spondyloarthropathy does not occur
(c) the joint disease is always symmetrical
(d) a symmetrical deforming polyarthropathy can occur
(e) most patients with arthropathy have a positive rheumatoid factor

### 11 Hypocomplementaemia occurs in the following
(a) essential mixed cryoglobulinaemia type 2
(b) infective endocarditis
(c) membranous nephropathy
(d) systemic lupus erythematosus
(e) mesangiocapillary glomerulonephritis

### 12 Antinuclear antibodies are
(a) very common in Sjögren's syndrome
(b) typical of systemic lupus erythematosus
(c) always clinically significant
(d) associated with iridocyclitis in juvenile arthritis

(e) present in most patients with rheumatoid arthritis

## 13 Antiphospholipid antibodies are associated with
(a) thrombocytopaenia
(b) a false positive antituberculin reaction
(c) thrombosis
(d) a positive lupus anticoagulant test
(e) a positive anticardiolipin test

## 14 Amyloidosis
(a) can complicate renal failure
(b) can cause renal failure
(c) is always caused by an underlying malignancy
(d) can be identified by isotope scanning
(e) occurs in familial Mediterranean fever

## 15 In the seronegative arthritides
(a) spondylitis is associated with HLA-B17
(b) there is always a history of a sexually transmitted disease
(c) positive rheumatoid factors are usual
(d) iritis only occurs with psoriatic arthropathy
(e) intervertebral disc calcification can occur

## 16 In the drug treatment of rheumatoid arthritis
(a) pencillamine can cause mesangiocapillary glomerulonephritis
(b) gold can cause nephrotic syndrome only if injected
(c) methotrexate therapy requires regular liver biopsy
(d) cyclophosphamide has a role
(e) there is no role for steroids

## 17 Of the nonsteroidal anti-inflammatory drugs
(a) ibuprofen is less nephrotoxic than diclofenac
(b) not all are associated with peptic ulceration
(c) there is no systemic absorption of topical preparations

(d) renal complications are more common in the young
(e) phenylbutazone is a well recognized cause of aplastic anaemia

## 18 In Paget's disease of bone
(a) the primary problem is excessive osteoblast activity
(b) urine phosphate can be diagnostic
(c) alkaline phosphatase is elevated
(d) diabetes insipidus is associated
(e) progression to sarcoma is usual

## 19 The following are true of osteoporosis
(a) it never occurs in men
(b) it occurs in Klinefelter's syndrome
(c) magnetic resonance imaging is the best routine form of assessment
(d) is usually associated with a raised alkaline phosphatase
(e) the amount of bone matrix is normal

## 20 Osteomalacia
(a) can be caused by chronic renal failure
(b) results from inadequate bone matrix
(c) can make standing up from a chair difficult
(d) is treated with 25-alpha-cholecalciferol in renal disease
(e) is usually associated with a low calcium and high phosphate if the kidneys are normal

# Mathematical medicine

## 1 Considering the following nine serum potassium values from different patients measured in mM: 2.5, 4, 3, 3, 3.5, 4, 6, 3, 7
(a) the median is 4 mM

(b) the mode is 6 mM
(c) the arithmetical mean is 5 mM
(d) if another set of values from different patients had a different standard deviation then the arithmetic mean must be different
(e) the standard deviation about the mean is 5 mM

## 2 The following statements are true

(a) the variance is the square root of the standard deviation
(b) the majority of a set of observations will be within two standard deviations of the arithmetic mean
(c) the standard deviation is inversely proportional to the dispersion of the sample data
(d) the population mean is always the same as the sample mean
(e) given only the standard deviation of a set of data the mean can be calculated

## 3 Considering the population from which a sample of heights are measured

(a) the population height can be predicted from the sample arithmetic mean and standard deviation
(b) the standard error of the mean is proportional to the square root of the sample size
(c) the standard error of the mean is proportional to the standard deviation of the sample
(d) the 95% confidence limits for the population mean get further apart as the standard error of the mean gets lower
(e) on average, 19 out of 20 times, the population height will be within the 95% confidence limits predicted by the sample data

**Questions** • Mathematical medicine

## 4 When comparing two samples of data from different groups
(a) Student's $t$ test is applicable to nonparametric data
(b) data with a normal distribution are suitable for parametric methods
(c) Kaplan–Meier analysis is ideal for nonparametric data
(d) the $t$ test assumes that the two samples have similar variances
(e) the F test can determine whether data is unsuitable for the $t$ test

## 5 When evaluating smoking as a risk factor for coronary heart disease
(a) the odds ratio for smokers cannot be calculated in a retrospective study of affected individuals
(b) case–control studies are of no benefit
(c) relative risk can be calculated from prospective studies
(d) confidence intervals can be calculated for odds ratios but not relative risks
(e) if the odds ratio for smokers was reduced then the risk of coronary disease in smokers would be increased

## 6 In an attempt to characterize a relationship between body weight and systolic blood pressure
(a) correlation analysis could be used
(b) regression analysis could be used
(c) the correlation coefficient measures the degree of association
(d) the correlation coefficient varies from 0 to 100
(e) linear regression can provide a quantitative expression linking the two variables

## 7 In analysing data from a clinical study
(a) multiple regression analysis can deal with more than three variables

(b) a $p$ value of 0.05 for a result means that there is a 1 in 19 chance that the result occurs by chance
(c) Chi square analysis is suitable for categorical data
(d) a scattergram is seldom of use in the analysis of an association between two variables
(e) the Mann–Whitney $U$ test is a nonparametric method to compare two independent groups

## 8 When designing a clinical trial of a new antithrombotic agent vs. placebo for the prevention of deep venous thrombosis in the postoperative period

(a) the power of the study will be greatest in a low risk group
(b) increasing the size of the study will increase the power
(c) a randomized controlled trial should be performed in preference to a case control study
(d) retrospective subgroup analysis is always reasonable in a randomized trial
(e) pilot studies may be necessary to determine the power of the main study

## 9 Considering a new diagnostic test for hepatitis C infection

(a) the sensitivity is the proportion of infected patients correctly identified by the test
(b) the specificity is the proportion of uninfected patients correctly identified by the test
(c) the negative predictive value is the proportion of patients with a negative test who are infected
(d) the positive predictive value is unaffected by the population prevalence of infection
(e) the likelihood ratio increases as the sensitivity of the test increases

**Questions** • Mathematical medicine

**10 In the analysis of survival from diagnosis of squamous cell carcinoma of the lung**

(a) Kaplan–Meier survival analysis can be applied

(b) the time of follow-up must be uniform for all patients in a Kaplan–Meier analysis

(c) Cox's proportional hazards analysis can be used to predict survival

(d) survival analysis of two groups treated in different ways will have wider confidence intervals as length of follow-up increases

(e) patients lost to follow-up after even half the study period can contribute nothing to a study using Kaplan–Meier analysis

# Answers

# Cardiology

### 1 F,F,T,T,F

The third heart sound occurs when there is a rush of blood into the ventricles in early diastole and is only normal under approximately 30 years of age. The fourth sound is caused by the ventricular filling associated with atrial systole and occurs in late ventricular diastole.

The jugular venous pulse (JVP) has two peaks and two descents following the peaks.

- The first or *a* peak represents atrial systole and is followed by the *x* descent representing downward movement of the heart during ventricular systole.
- The second or *v* peak reflects venous return into the right atrium during ventricular systole and is followed by the *y* descent representing a fall, in pressure with the opening of the tricuspid valve between the right atrium and right ventricle.

The height of the jugular venous pulse is a reflection of right atrial pressure and should fall on inspiration as the chest expands and intrathoracic pressure falls. A rise on inspiration suggests pericardial constriction (Kussmaul's sign). The pulse rate can be slightly faster in inspiration than expiration, this is a normal occurrence and is known as sinus arrhythmia. A dicrotic notch is a normal finding and is a slight dip in the peak of the carotid pulse which occurs when the aortic valve closes.

### 2 T,T,F,T,T

The QT interval on the electrocardiograph is measured from the onset of the QRS complex to the end of the T wave and reflects ventricular repolarization. The QTc is the QT interval corrected for heart rate.

**Answers** • Cardiology

- Mutations in the *LQT3 SCN5A* gene on chromosome 3 and in the *LQT2 HERG* gene on chromosome 7 can both result in a prolonged QT syndrome. The *LQT3 SCN5A* gene encodes a potassium channel and the *LQT2 HERG* gene encodes a sodium channel.
- Hypocalcaemia prolongs the QTc interval and hypercalcaemia shortens it.
- The Romano–Ward syndrome is an autosomal dominant condition causing prolongation of the QTc interval.
- The Jervell–Lange–Nielsen syndrome is an autosomal recessive condition with deafness and a long QTc.
- Quinidine is a class 1a antiarrhythmic and so prolongs the QTc interval, lignocaine is a class 1b antiarrhythmic and so does not prolong the QTc interval.

**3 T,T,T,F,T**

Normally the aortic valve closes before the pulmonary valve. This is because of the higher pressure acting to close it in the systemic arterial system compared to the pressure in the pulmonary artery acting on the pulmonary valve. In aortic stenosis, it takes longer for the ventricle to empty against the stenosed valve, so aortic valve closure is delayed and may occur after pulmonary valve closure. This is known as a reversed split. Mitral regurgitation lowers left ventricular pressure during systole and so the aortic valve closes early widening the normal split. Right bundle branch block delays right ventricular contraction and can widen the normal split between the aortic valve closure and pulmonary valve closure. Inspiration expands the chest, lowering the pressure in the pulmonary arterial tree. The resistance to flow out of the right ventricle is reduced and the pulmonary valve closes even later than normal so widening the normal split. A patent ductus arteriosus joins the pulmonary artery to the aorta and so pulmonary arterial pressure is high causing

Cardiology • **Answers**

early closure of the pulmonary valve and so a reversed split. The pulmonary valve closes first with a patent ductus as right ventricular pressure is lower than left because the right ventricle is initially weaker than the left.

## 4 T,T,F,T,F

The distinction between hyperkalaemia and hypokalaemia is critical. Both hypokalaemia and hyperkalaemia are associated with dysrhythmias. A particularly dangerous association is ventricular tachycardia or fibrillation resulting from hyperkalaemia.

- The typical changes of hyperkalaemia on the ECG are progressive loss of P waves, widening of the QRS complex, loss of the S–T segment and tall wide T waves. As the potassium level rises, these changes produce an almost sine wave appearance.
- The typical changes of hypokalaemia are progressive lengthening of the PR interval, S–T segment depression, loss of the T wave and an increase in the U wave.

## 5 T,T,F,F,F

Constrictive pericarditis is usually a chronic condition with a fibrotic pericardium. As a consequence, the jugular venous pressure (JVP) is usually elevated and rises on inspiration, an abnormality known as Kussmaul's sign. Under normal circumstances, the JVP falls on inspiration because thoracic pressure falls and the heart is distensible; the fall in intrathoracic pressure also encourages venous return. However, in constrictive pericarditis, there is increased venous return during inspiration to a nondistensible heart and so the jugular venous pressure rises. A pericardial knock may occur which is a third heart sound formed when there is rapid ventricular filling of the indistensible ventricles in early diastole. Pulsus paradoxus is a larger than normal fall in pulse pressure on inspiration.

## Answers • Cardiology

- Pulsus paradoxus is uncommon in constrictive pericarditis, but is always present in cardiac tamponade.
- In constrictive pericarditis, both the $x$ and $y$ descents of the JVP become prominent, but in tamponade only the $x$ descent is prominent and the $y$ descent is often lost.

The management of constrictive pericarditis involves the treatment of any underlying disorder such as tuberculosis and, if possible, surgery to remove the pericardium. Urgent needle aspiration is only necessary in the presence of life threatening cardiac tamponade caused by pericardial fluid.

### 6 T,F,F,F,F

The main cardiac causes of cyanosis at birth are:
- transposition of the great arteries (TGA);
- severe pulmonary stenosis;
- hypoplasia of the left heart;
- tricuspid atresia;
- pulmonary atresia;
- a severe Ebstein's anomaly with an atrial septal defect (ASD).

Any right to left shunt bypasses the lungs and can cause cyanosis. Obstructions to right ventricular outflow such as pulmonary stenosis can cause high right-sided pressure and a right to left shunt through a patent foramen ovale. The foramen ovale is open in 25% of otherwise normal births. A patent ductus arteriosus joins the pulmonary artery to the aorta and initially causes a left to right shunt because the left-sided pressure is higher. Similarly, an atrial septal defect initially causes a left to right shunt between the atria. A large ventricular septal defect initially causes a left to right shunt between the ventricles. Ebstein's anomaly is atrialization of the right ventricle, with the result that part of what would normally be the atrium is in the ventricle. The right ventricle is weak so right ventricular end diastolic pressure is high, and as tricuspid regurgitation often occurs, an ASD will allow a right to left shunt in Ebstein's anomaly.

## 7 T,F,T,T,T

The cardiac action potential (see Fig. 1) is complex, but certain points are important. The electrical potential across the cell membrane is determined not only by the ionic concentration gradient across the membrane, but also by how permeable the membrane is to the these ions. In electrical terms, the

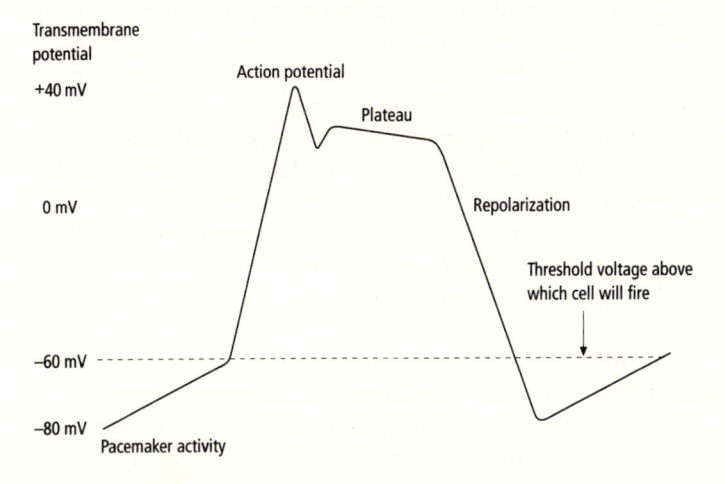

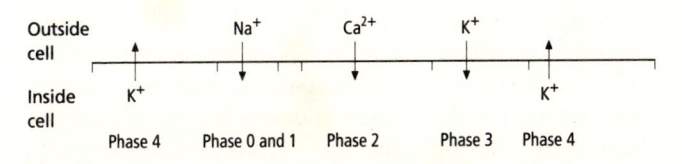

**Figure 1** The cardiac action potential. Changes in transmembrane potential are determined by ion flow across the cell membrane. Changes in the conductance for different ions reflect changes in the ion channels in the cell membrane.

## Answers • Cardiology

permeability is expressed as conductance. Outside the cell the concentration of sodium is high and potassium low; inside the cell the concentration of sodium is low and potassium high.

- At rest the membrane is impermeable to sodium and calcium, but permeable to potassium. This means that potassium can flow across the membrane and so the conductance for potassium is high. Thus, potassium levels determines the baseline resting potential and abnormalities of potassium can cause abnormal cardiac rhythms.
- On depolarization, which occurs spontaneously in cells with intrinsic pacemaker activity, sodium permeability or conductance increases dramatically and the membrane potential becomes positive as sodium ions enter the cell. Calcium ions flow in during the plateau phase of the action potential keeping the membrane potential positive for longer.

Lignocaine is a local anaesthetic and antiarrhythmic of class 1b action. Such drugs can reduce sodium conductance and so reduce the excitability of cardiac tissue.

### 8 F,F,F,T,F

Platelets produce thromboxanes which promote platelet aggregation and clot formation; the vascular endothelium produces prostacyclins which oppose this. Aspirin non-selectively blocks cyclo-oxygenase, an enzyme involved in the synthesis of both prostacyclins and thromboxanes from their arachidonic acid precursors in both endothelium and platelets. An irreversible acetylation of the enzyme occurs in both platelets and the endothelium, but unlike the endothelium, the platelets cannot synthesise new enzymes as they have no nuclear apparatus. Platelets are, therefore, affected most and this reduces the risk of thrombosis in many settings by reducing platelet aggregation. In large properly conducted trials, such as the ISIS 2 trial, aspirin given following myocardial infarction reduces both mortality and reinfarction (*Lancet* 1988; **2**: 349–60). When clearly indicated, it can be used at low doses in renal failure with care and with careful monitoring for adverse reactions. There is no need for routine ulcer prophylaxis if aspirin is given with thrombolysis post myocardial infarction.

## 9 F,T,F,T,T

In mitral stenosis, the first heart sound is loud, as the mitral valve stays open throughout ventricular diastole and is suddenly shut by ventricular systole. As the stenosed valve opens during ventricular diastole there is a snap which gets nearer to the second heart sound as the severity increases. This occurs to maximize the time available for flow through the narrowed valve. The characteristic diastolic murmur is caused by this flow. Because of the obstruction to left atrial outflow, left atrial pressure is raised. Pulmonary arterial wedge pressure reflects left atrial pressure and is therefore also elevated. The high left atrial pressures are conveyed to the pulmonary vascular tree and chronic pulmonary arterial hypertension with right ventricular hypertrophy can occur as a result. Haemoptysis can be caused by bronchial vein rupture, pulmonary oedema, infection or infarction. Digoxin is used only to control established atrial fibrillation. Anti-coagulation prevents thrombus formation, especially in the left atrium when there is atrial fibrillation. This is important, as systemic emboli from the heart are a cause of serious morbidity mainly from stroke.

## 10 F,F,T,F,T

Any cause of myocardial dysfunction can result in the syndrome of congestive heart failure. Ischaemic heart disease is the commonest in Europe, but chronic Chagas' disease caused by *Trypanosomiasis cruzi* is an important cause in the

## Answers • Cardiology

American continent. In congestive heart failure, there is weakness of ventricular contraction resulting in reduced cardiac output. In addition, ventricular relaxation is often abnormal. The normal left ventricular end diastolic pressure is around 12–15 mmHg but this may rise to 30 mmHg in left ventricular failure. In heart failure, various reflexes are associated with the low cardiac output. There is increased sympathetic tone, increased antidiuretic hormone (ADH) production and activation of the renin-angiotensin-aldosterone system. There are also enhanced levels of the vasoconstrictor endothelin 1. The key results of these reflexes are sodium conservation by the kidney and increased peripheral resistance due to increased peripheral vessel tone. Therapy aims to oppose these actions with vasodilators, diuretics and angiotensin converting enzyme inhibitors.

## 11 F,T,F,T,T

Epidemiological studies show that the risk of coronary heart disease is proportional to serum total cholesterol. The normal range for a population is defined as being within two standard deviations of the population mean. Although 4.5 mmol is within the normal range for the UK, there is still a significant risk of heart disease at this level, as the normal range is defined for a population which already has a substantial risk. The lower the cholesterol, the lower the risk. The ratio in serum of HDL:LDL (high density and low density lipoprotein) cholesterol seems important, with a lower risk associated with a greater proportion of total cholesterol in the form of HDL cholesterol.

• Left anterior descending artery thrombosis causes anterior infarction; right coronary artery thrombosis causes inferior infarction.

• The right coronary artery usually supplies the atrioventricular node as well as the inferior ventricle.

Ischaemia of the atrioventricular node can cause heart block during an inferior infarction, but as the node is also supplied by the left coronary artery system, recovery is usual. In anterior infarction, heart block usually represents damage to the left bundle branches which have no right sided blood supply and so recovery is not as likely and pacing is usually necessary. This usually occurs with a large anterior infarction and carries a poor prognosis.

Multiple prethrombolysis trials, such as the ISIS 1 trial (*Lancet* 1986; **2**: 57–66), showed reduced mortality with the use of beta blockers, but these results preceded those involving angiotensin converting enzyme inhibitors in acute myocardial infarction and there are no clear comparisons of beta blockade and angiotensin converting enzyme inhibition. Beta blockers may act by an antiarrhythmic effect or by reducing myocardial oxygen consumption and so progressive infarction in the ischaemic peri-infarct zone.

## 12 T,T,T,F,T

Q wave infarction usually results from occlusion of a main coronary artery and subsequent infarction of the region of the ventricle supplied by the artery. In contrast, non-Q wave infarctions represent lesser degrees of myocardial damage, often due to incomplete occlusion of the artery by atherosclerotic plaque or thrombus or both. The pathophysiology is illustrated in Fig. 2.

Because of ventricular contraction, a gradient exists within the ventricular wall with intramural pressure increasing from the surface to the ventricular cavity. The coronary arteries supply blood from the outside, so there is a pressure gradient in the myocardium opposing blood flow. If the pressure head in the coronary arteries is reduced because of an upstream obstruction, the area most vulnerable to ischaemia is the inside of the ventricular wall, the subendocardium. This can cause a non-Q wave or subendocardial infarction and

## Answers • Cardiology

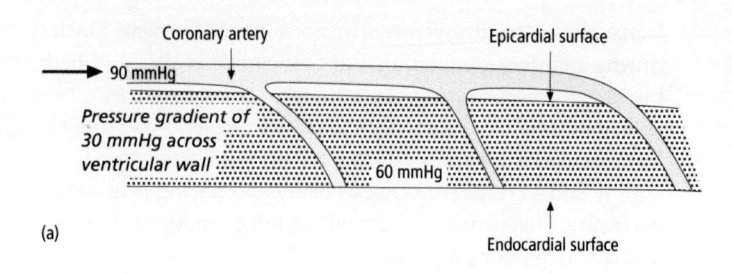

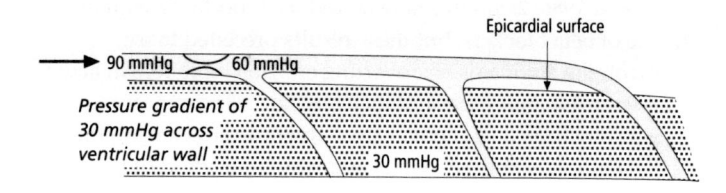

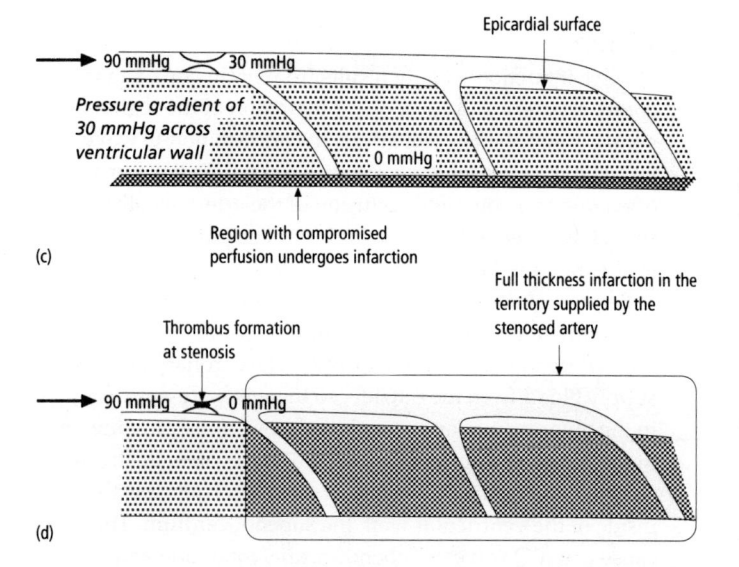

(a) Coronary artery → 90 mmHg, Epicardial surface, Pressure gradient of 30 mmHg across ventricular wall, 60 mmHg, Endocardial surface

(b) 90 mmHg → 60 mmHg, Epicardial surface, Pressure gradient of 30 mmHg across ventricular wall, 30 mmHg

(c) 90 mmHg → 30 mmHg, Epicardial surface, Pressure gradient of 30 mmHg across ventricular wall, 0 mmHg, Region with compromised perfusion undergoes infarction

(d) Thrombus formation at stenosis, 90 mmHg → 0 mmHg, Full thickness infarction in the territory supplied by the stenosed artery

although the initial damage is often minimal, the upstream stenosis remains and can occlude completely to produce a full thickness transmural Q wave infarct. For this reason early mortality is low, but reinfarction is common and early investigation, preferably before discharge, is mandatory to detect and treat any stenoses. Diltiazem has been shown to improve outcome in non-Q wave infarction.

### 13 F,F,T,T,F

The key risk factors for thoracic aortic dissection are:
- hypertension;
- Marfan's syndrome;
- coarctation of the aorta.

Homocystinuria is not associated with aortic dissection, but it can present with a similar phenotype to Marfan's syndrome. Syphilis causes aortic aneurysms, which may rupture, but do not usually dissect. Ankylosing spondylitis is associated with aortic valve regurgitation.

### 14 T,F,F,F,T

The key aspect about a ventricular tachycardia is that the atrioventricular node does not usually conduct backwards, so it may be possible to identify independent atrial activity which is not under the influence of the abnormal ventricular pacemaker.
- Cannon waves occur in the jugular venous pulse when the

---

**Figure 2** (*Left.*) Non-Q-wave infarcts. (a) Normally there is a drop in the arterial pressure as the arteries descend into the myocardium. (b) If a stenosis develops this reduces the arterial pressure distal to it. (c) If the stenosis becomes severe, then the arterial pressure distal to it can no longer perfuse the entire thickness of the myocardium and infarction of the inner wall can occur. (d) If the stenosis worsens still further and blocks the artery, by for example thrombus formation, then a full thickness infarct of all the supplied myocardium can occur.

## Answers • Cardiology

atria and ventricle contract independently as the atrium contracts against a closed tricuspid valve.
• Fusion beats occur on the ECG when a normal atrial impulse travels down the atrioventricular node and joins with the ventricular impulse to produce a single different QRS complex.
• Capture beat occur in the ECG when a normal atrial impulse causes a normal QRS complex for one beat during a ventricular rhythm. Usually only supra-ventricular tachycardias respond to adenosine.

### 15 T,T,T,T,T

Aortic ring dilatation resulting in aortic valve regurgitation occurs in:
• syphilis;
• relapsing polychondritis;
• osteogenesis imperfecta;
• the seronegative arthritides, such as ankylosing spondylitis.

In infective endocarditis, infection of the valve causes mechanical inadequacy of valve closure and so regurgitation.

### 16 T,T,F,F,T

Left posterior hemiblock is block of the posterior branch of the left bundle branch and is associated with right axis deviation. In contrast, block of the anterior branch of the left bundle branch is known as left anterior hemiblock and is associated with left axis deviation. A primum atrial septal defect (ASD) can be associated with left axis deviation whereas a secundum defect is associated with right axis deviation. The strain imposed on the right ventricle by a partially occluded pulmonary vasculature in the context of a pulmonary embolus can produce right axis deviation as can any cause of pulmonary hypertension.

Cardiology • **Answers**

## 17 F,T,T,T,F

In first degree heart block there is a delay in conduction through the atrioventricular node. In third degree heart block there is no conduction through the node, whereas in second degree, some, but not all atrial impulses are conducted. A complete or partial block to atrioventricular nodal conduction can slow the ventricular rate, but delayed conduction across the atrioventricular node does not in itself slow the pulse. For this reason, first degree block causes lengthening of the P-R interval on an ECG because of delayed atrioventricular nodal conduction, but by itself does not slow heart rate. When there is complete or third degree heart block across the atrioventricular node, the slow intrinsic pacemakers in the ventricle control the ventricular and so the pulse rate.

Normally, heart rate is determined by the pacemaker action of the sino-atrial node. In sick sinus syndrome, sino-atrial block can occur between the sinus node itself and the atrium causing bradycardia. Sick sinus syndrome can also result in tachycardia if there is dysfunctional sino-atrial node over-activity. Digoxin can block atrioventricular nodal conduction thus slowing heart rate. Bradycardia is typical of the general metabolic slowing of hypothyroidism. In raised intracranial pressure, there is reflex bradycardia. Bradycardia is not a feature of Gaucher's disease which is a sex-linked recessive lysosomal storage disease.

## 18 T,F,T,T,F

In the Wolff–Parkinson–White syndrome an aberrant conduction pathway known as the bundle of Kent permits fast conduction of atrial impulses to the ventricles so shortening the P-R interval and producing delta waves on the upstroke of the QRS complex. The two main rhythms are re-entrant supraventricular tachycardia and atrial fibrillation, the latter occurring less commonly. Digoxin and the class 4

## Answers • Cardiology

antiarrhythmics which are calcium antagonists, such as verapamil, can further increase the speed of conduction down the bundle of Kent. In atrial fibrillation, such an increase can allow a dangerously fast ventricular rate to occur resulting in haemodynamic collapse.

- In type A, the accessory pathway is on the left side of the heart and this produces a positive QRS in V1.
- In type B, the accessory pathway is on the right side and the QRS is usually negative in V1.

### 19 F,T,F,F,F

The principal adrenergic receptor types are alpha-1, alpha-2, beta-1 and beta-2. Of the beta receptors, beta-1 receptors in the heart mediate positive inotropism and beta-2 receptors in the lungs mediate bronchodilation. Alpha-receptors mediate systemic vasoconstriction. Adrenaline acts on all these receptors and is a powerful inotrope. Dobutamine is a beta-1 selective agonist and so a positive inotrope. Isoprenaline is a nonspecific beta-agonist with no significant alpha-agonist activity. Salbutamol is a selective beta-2-agonist, but not a beta-1 blocker. Dopamine is a positive inotrope with beta-1 and alpha agonist activity at high doses; it also has actions at lower doses on separate dopaminergic receptors which increase renal and mesenteric blood flow.

### 20 T,T,T,T,T

Sudden death may occur in around 7.5% of cases of aortic stenosis. Atrioventricular block can occur if calcification of the aortic ring extends into the upper ventricular septum damaging the conducting system. Bicuspid valves occur in 1% of the population, but do not always cause aortic stenosis. During ventricular systole, the high pressure within the myocardium prevents effective flow of blood to the muscle from the coronary arteries, so most of the flow is in diastole. As aortic stenosis develops, systole is prolonged and the

Cardiology/Endocrinology • **Answers**

ventricular pressure increased, which increases the myocardial oxygen requirement. Unfortunately, diastole is shortened and so myocardial blood flow and oxygen delivery is reduced. The gradient across the valve during systole increases with increasing severity of the stenosis.

# Endocrinology

## 1 T,T,T,T,F

In simple terms, cholesterol is converted to pregnenolone then progesterone. Both these products can give rise to cortisol, aldosterone or testosterone. Testosterone can be converted in the ovaries to oestrogens. 5-alpha-reductase converts testosterone to dihydrotestosterone – both products being androgens. Finasteride is a 5-alpha-reductase inhibitor and is used in the treatment of prostatic hypertrophy which is androgen related. 5-alpha-reductase deficiency results in an undervirilized male baby, but has no obvious effect on women. Congenital adrenal hyperplasia results in over-virilization of female babies and occurs when there is a deficiency in an enzyme in the steroid synthetic pathway, usually 21 hydroxylase. As there is a drive to produce more steroids, this results in excess testosterone and dihydrotestosterone which are not affected by the 21 hydroxylase deficiency. The various pathways of steroid biosynthesis are shown in Fig. 3.

## 2 T,T,T,T,T

In acute liver failure deficient maintenance of blood glucose results from impaired liver function includin glycogenolysis. Steroids help to maintain blood glucose, particularly by stimulating glucose production by the liver and deficiency in Addison's disease is associated with a low blood glucose

## Answers • Endocrinology

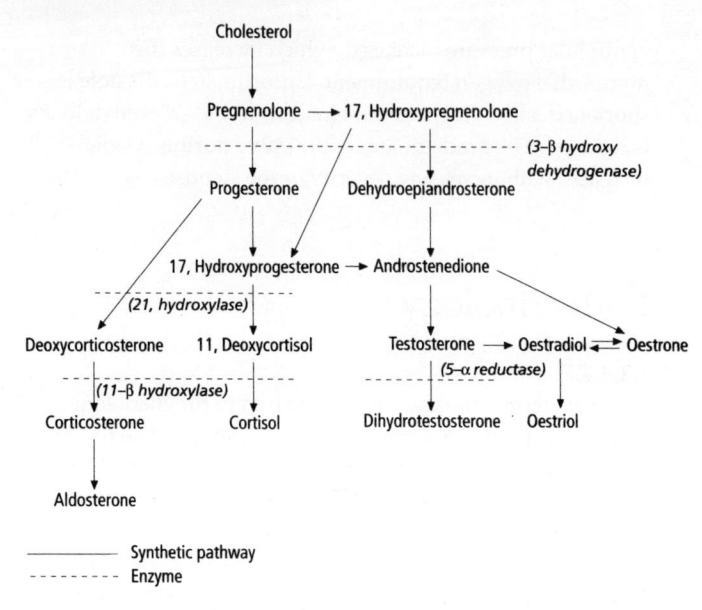

**Figure 3** The steroid biosynthetic pathways.

level. Sulphonylureas have a hypoglycaemic effect as their principal action by increasing insulin sensitivity. The glycogen storage diseases are all recessive and result in the storage of excess glycogen or abnormally structured glycogen in tissues. The pathology reflects the organs in which this occurs and the main types and their features are:

- Type I (von Gierke): hepatomegaly, hypoglycaemia, hypotonia, obesity and poor growth;
- Type II (Pompe): cardiomyopathy and heart failure resulting in death in infancy;
- Type III (Forbes): hepatomegaly, hypoglycaemia – a mild form of type I;
- Type IV (Anderson): hepatomegaly, cirrhosis and portal hypertension;
- Type V (McArdle): skeletal muscle cramps, fatigue and myoglobinuria.

## 3 T,T,T,F,T

Growth hormone has a diurnal cycle with a rise at night. Intuitively, this makes sense providing for growth and consolidation during the rest period of the diurnal cycle. Usually a glucose tolerance test suppresses growth hormone levels, but in acromegaly there is no suppression. The glucose tolerance test is itself often abnormal in acromegaly, with around a quarter of acromegalic patients having a diabetic profile. Acromegaly results from growth hormone excess and can cause tissue growth and expansion leading to carpal tunnel syndrome.

## 4 T,F,F,T,T

The common causes of hyperthyroidism are:
- Graves disease which is associated with thyroid-stimulating antibodies;
- toxic nodular goitres;
- thyroiditis.

A low TSH (thyroid stimulating hormone) is consistent with hyperthyroidism, but serum thyroxine (T4) can be normal if serum triiodothyronine (T3) levels are high. In pregnancy and in women on the contraceptive pill, thyroxine binding globulin (TBG) levels are often high and total thyroxine levels may be elevated, although free thyroxine levels are normal. A rise in TSH on administration of thyrotrophin-releasing hormone (TRH) does not occur in hyperthyroidism due to feedback suppression on TSH by thyroxine or triiodothyronine. Carbimazole reduces the production of thyroid hormones by inhibiting the iodination of thyroglobulin. Adverse effects of the drug include a rash and agranulocytosis.

## 5 T,T,T,T,T

The main endocrine causes of a proximal myopathy are:
- vitamin D deficiency;

## Answers • Endocrinology

- excess corticosteroids;
- excess growth hormone;
- thyrotoxicosis.

Vitamin D deficiency causes osteomalacia and a proximal myopathy. Excess endogenous or exogenous corticosteroid can cause a proximal myopathy, as can acromegaly and polymyositis. Duchenne muscular dystrophy is associated with a proximal muscle weakness whereas dystrophia myotonica is associated with distal weakness as well as cataracts, frontal baldness and cardiomyopathies.

### 6 T,F,T,T,F

The key feature of polycystic ovary syndrome is that there is defective synthesis of oestradiol in the ovaries with accumulation of precursors which can be converted to oestrone and testosterone in tissues outside the ovary. The syndrome is therefore associated with excess androgen production and luteinising hormone levels are usually raised with respect to follicle stimulating hormone. Typically, 3–5 mm cysts are seen on ultrasound examination. Common clinical findings are obesity, amenorrhoea or oligomenorrhoea, infertility and hirsutism.

### 7 T,T,T,F,T

Both exogenous or endogenous excess of steroid hormones is associated with osteoporosis. Sex hormone deficiencies, whether resulting from primary hypogonadism or the post-menopausal state are associated with osteoporosis. Heparin, given for a prolonged period of time, such as during pregnancy for valvular heart disease, can cause osteoporosis. The reasons for osteoporosis in rheumatoid arthritis are not clear and may relate to immobility, therapy and the chronic inflammatory nature of disease itself.

Endocrinology • **Answers**

**8** T,T,T,F,T

Polyuria can result from inadequate antidiuretic hormone action, impaired tubular reabsorption of water in the kidney or excess water intake. Hypercalcaemia and acute tubular necrosis interfere with tubular function, thus promoting water loss in the kidney. Lithium can cause nephrogenic diabetes insipidus with an inadequate renal response to antidiuretic hormone. Chlorpropamide, in contrast, can cause a syndrome of inappropriate excess antidiuretic hormone (SIADH) with inappropriate water conservation.

**9** T,T,F,T,T

Prolactin normally promotes lactation, but excess can cause galactorrhoea and infertility. The hypothalamus synthesizes dopamine which is an inhibitor of prolactin secretion, so dopamine antagonists such as phenothiazines can block this normal inhibition causing hyperprolactinaemia. Bromocriptine is a dopamine agonist and so inhibits prolactin secretion. In acromegaly raised levels of prolactin are not uncommon.

**10** F,F,T,F,T

Testicular feminization syndrome occurs when there is a deficiency of androgens. The classic disease is X-linked and is associated with various mutations in testosterone receptors, though testosterone itself is normal. As the disease is X-linked, males are affected and testosterone levels are high. However, because of the receptor defect they are phenotypically female. At puberty, female secondary sexual characteristics develop as a result of oestradiol. Infertility occurs. A similar syndrome can occur if there is a defect in testosterone production.

**11** T,T,T,T,T

The Diabetes Control and Complication trial demonstrated

## Answers • Endocrinology

that tight glycaemic control delayed the onset and progression of retinopathy, nephropathy and neuropathy (*New England Journal of Medicine* 1994: **329**; 977–86). The main adverse effect was a two to threefold increase in severe hypoglycaemia. Blood pressure control with angiotensin converting enzyme inhibitors seems to slow the progression of nephropathy. Nephropathy is usually associated with retinopathy.

### 12 F,F,T,T,T

In noninsulin dependent diabetes mellitus (NIDDM) there is peripheral resistance to the effects of insulin and ultimately reduced insulin secreting capacity in response to hyperglycaemia. The key aspect of management is to reduce weight as 75% of patients are obese at presentation and to use foods that release carbohydrate slowly, such as pasta, as these aid glycaemic control.

- Sulphonylureas stimulate insulin secretion from beta cells in the pancreas and may enhance some of the actions of insulin such as the inhibition of hepatic glucose production. Sulphonylureas can cause hypoglycaemia.
- Biguanides, such as metformin, reduce hepatic glucose production and intestinal glucose absorption, but do not cause insulin secretion and do not cause hypoglycaemia. Metformin is renally excreted and an accumulation can cause lactic acidosis.
- Acarbose is an alpha glucosidase inhibitor and reduces intestinal glucose absorption so reducing post-prandial hyperglycaemia and helping the maintenance of euglycaemia.

### 13 T,F,F,T,F

Parathyroid hormone causes renal phosphate excretion via a cyclic adenosine monophosphate (cAMP) mediated mechanism and increases bone resorption by osteoclasts.

Usually this is accompanied by renal conservation of calcium and serum calcium rises and serum phosphate falls. The principal trigger to parathyroid hormone secretion is the serum calcium level, with a low serum calcium increasing secretion and a high serum calcium suppressing secretion.
- In primary hypoparathyroidism there is excessive parathyroid hormone secretion resulting in hypercalcaemia.
- In contrast, in secondary hyperparathyroidism the serum calcium is low and the excessive parathyroid hormone secretion is an appropriate response to attempt to correct the low calcium.
- Tertiary hyperparathyroidism can occur following secondary hyperparathyroidism if the parathyroid glands become autonomous and continue to secrete excess hormone even when serum calcium is normal.

The metabolic changes in renal bone disease are complex and variable, but there is often excess parathyroid hormone secretion and deficient vitamin D synthesis. The kidney normally excretes phosphate. In renal disease phosphate accumulates and calcium may initially fall, stimulating parathyroid hormone secretion which may ultimately become autonomous (tertiary hyper-parathyroidism). Renal damage reduces the capacity of the kidney to produce the active vitamin D metabolite 1,25-dihydroxycholecalciferol. Cholecalciferol (vitamin $D_3$) is produced in the skin by photoactivation of 7-dehydrocholesterol. The liver converts this to 25-hydroxycholecalciferol and the kidney converts this to 1,25-dihydroxycholecalciferol. The steps in vitamin D synthesis are illustrated in Fig. 4.

## 14 T,T,T,T,T

The hypothalamus secretes corticotrophin releasing factor (CRF) which causes secretion of adrenocorticotrophic hormone (ACTH) from the pituitary. ACTH triggers the release of corticosteroid from the zona fasciculata and zona

## Answers • Endocrinology

reticularis of the adrenal cortex. Cushing's disease is the result of an ACTH producing pituitary adenoma. Cushing's syndrome typically describes the phenotype resulting from excess corticosteroid, regardless of the aetiology. Cortisol has many actions, but in particular it triggers hepatic gluconeogenesis and hepatic glycogen production and may reduce peripheral glucose utilization. In the kidney, there is a mineralocorticoid effect which increases sodium conservation, but can, in excess, result in hypokalaemia.

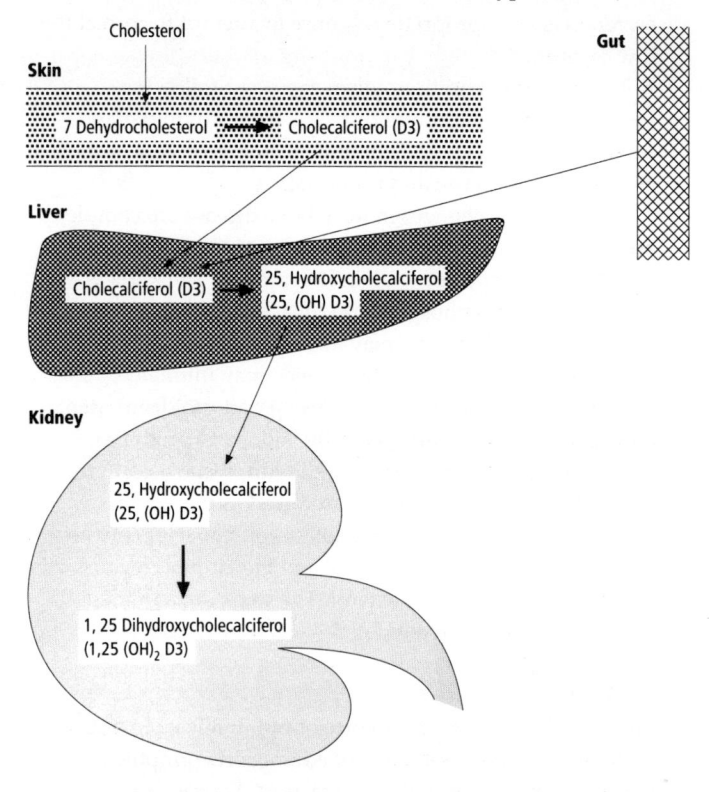

**Figure 4** Vitamin D synthesis.

Lowered blood glucose normally triggers cortisol secretion and this is the principle underlying the insulin stress test. In contrast, dexamethasone normally inhibits secretion and this is the basis for the dexamethasone suppression test. Steroid levels are higher during the day and this facilitates the maintenance of blood glucose levels during the active period of the daily cycle.

## 15 T,F,T,T,F

Unopposed oestrogens reduce the risk of bone fractures and coronary artery disease and improve lipid profiles after the menopause. However, unopposed oestrogens increase the risk of endometrial cancer, but this effect is virtually eliminated by cyclical progestogen treatment. There may be a slightly increased risk of breast cancer with prolonged hormone treatment and a number of recent studies have shown an increased incidence of venous thrombosis.

## 16 T,F,T,F,T

A phaeochromocytoma is a tumour which secretes catecholamines and can arise anywhere in the sympathetic-adrenal system from the neck to the pelvis. However, most tumours arise in the adrenal medulla. Clinical features include palpitation, tremor, headache, chest pain and sometimes postural hypotension. A myocarditis can occur and may be fatal. Vanillylmandelic acid (VMA) is a metabolite of catecholamines and levels are usually raised. 5-hydroxyindoleacetic acid (5-HIAA) is a serotonin metabolite and may be raised in the carcinoid syndrome. Alpha blockade is given before beta blockade, to prevent an unopposed alpha-adrenergic effect on the cardiovascular system which can result in severe hypertension. The main associated conditions are neurofibromatosis and multiple endocrine neoplasia (MEN) type IIa.

**Answers** • Endocrinology

### 17 T,T,T,T,F

Diabetic autonomic neuropathy is common, but often asymptomatic. Features include impaired gastric emptying, altered gut hormone responses to meals, diminished cardiovascular reflexes with postural hypotension and impaired Valsalva heart rate responses. Bladder dysfunction with urinary retention is rare but can occur.

### 18 F,T,F,F,F

Hyperthyroidism is unusual with thyroid cancer. The principle tumours are papillary, follicular, medullary, anaplastic and lymphoma. The commonest by far is the papillary tumour which is slow growing and occurs particularly in the young. Follicular and papillary tumours have a good prognosis if treated, whereas anaplastic and medullary cell tumours carry a poor prognosis. Typically, follicular tumours occur in late middle age, with anaplastic tumours arising in the elderly. Medullary tumours arise from the C cells which produce calcitonin and may be associated with multiple endocrine neoplasia syndromes.

### 19 T,T,T,T,F

Many changes occur in pregnancy including a rise in heart rate, renal blood flow and glomerular filtration rate. The rise in glomerular filtration rate is associated with a fall in serum urea and creatinine. Prolactin levels rise which prepares the breasts for lactation. As there is no menstrual cycle, the secretion of luteinising hormone and follicular stimulating hormone is inhibited during pregnancy.

### 20 T,T,T,T,T

In Klinefelter's syndrome the karyotype is XXY chromosomes, whereas in Turner's syndrome it is XO. Both conditions are associated with infertility. The phenotype in Klinefelter's syndrome is male with female secondary sexual characteristics. The phenotype in Turner's syndrome is female with short stature, a low hairline, a shield chest with widely shaped nipples and poorly developed secondary sexual characteristics. There are associations in Turner's syndrome with coarctation of the aorta, renal anomalies – such as horseshoe kidneys, autoimmune thyroiditis and diabetes mellitus. Any cause of hyperprolactinaemia can cause infertility as prolactin appears to alter the normal feedback control of oestrogen on luteinising and follicular stimulating hormones.

# Gastroenterology

## 1 T,T,T,T,T

*Helicobacter pylori* is present in almost all cases of antral gastritis and is likely to play a role in the pathogenesis of this gastritis. Most patients with duodenal ulceration also have chronic antral gastritis and eradication of *H. pylori* is associated with long-term ulcer cure. There is an association between carriage of the organism and gastric ulceration, but it is not as strong for gastric as for duodenal ulceration. Both gastric mucosa associated lymphoid tissue (MALT) lymphoma and gastric adenocarcinoma are associated with *H. pylori* and eradication of the organism has been associated with remission of gastric MALT lymphoma.

## 2 T,T,T,T,T

Malabsorption results in generalized malnutrition and weight loss and can be caused by disease of the pancreas or bowel. Fat malabsorption causes steatorrhoea. There may, in addition, be deficiencies of vitamins, especially the fat soluble vitamins A, D and E. Vitamin D deficiency can contribute to a serum low calcium concentration. Vitamin K deficiency may cause abnormal clotting and thiamine (vitamin $B_1$) deficiency can result in neuropathy.

### 3 T,T,F,T,T

The three well recognized mediators of increased gastric acid secretion are gastrin, histamine (acting through $H_2$ receptors) and acetylcholine which can be blocked by atropine. Both atropine and histamine antagonists reduce the acid secretory response to gastrin. Glucagon is mainly produced by alpha cells in the pancreas and stimulates glycogenolysis and the maintenance of blood glucose. Vasoactive intestinal peptide (VIP) can occur in excess with VIPomas which are associated with secretory diarrhoea.

### 4 T,T,T,T,T

The commonest cause of acute pancreatitis is gallstones and the next commonest is alcohol. Poor prognostic features include advanced age, and markers of sepsis or multi-organ dysfunction such as hypoxia, renal failure, hyperglycaemia, hypoalbuminaemia, hypocalcaemia, liver dysfunction and a raised white cell count. In the presence of impacted gallstones early endoscopy and stone removal is of benefit. Other therapeutic strategies such as the use of octreotide to inhibit pancreatic secretion may be of benefit but are still being evaluated. Purtscher's angiopathic retinopathy is a rare complication with flame-shaped haemorrhages and cotton-wool spots and can cause sudden blindness.

### 5 T,T,T,T,T

Most infected individuals are either intravenous drug users or recipients of contaminated blood, but mother to infant transmission can occur. In an ELISA (enzyme linked immunosorbent assay), antibodies are used to detect the presence of a specific protein and an enzyme attached to the antibodies can be used to produce a colour change which is easily measured spectrophotometrically. Although ELISA is a highly sensitive diagnostic test, it may take up to 6 months for an antibody response to develop after primary infection and in immunosuppressed individuals there may be no detectable antibody response. For these reasons, the most sensitive diagnostic rather than screening test is PCR (polymerase chain reaction) amplification of cDNA. cDNA is made by reverse transcription of mRNA. The principles of the ELISA and PCR methods of diagnosis are shown in Figs 5 and 6, respectively.

## 6 T,F,T,T,F

The key risk factors for non-steroidal anti-inflammatory drug (NSAID) induced gastrointestinal problems are:
- age;
- alcohol related disease;

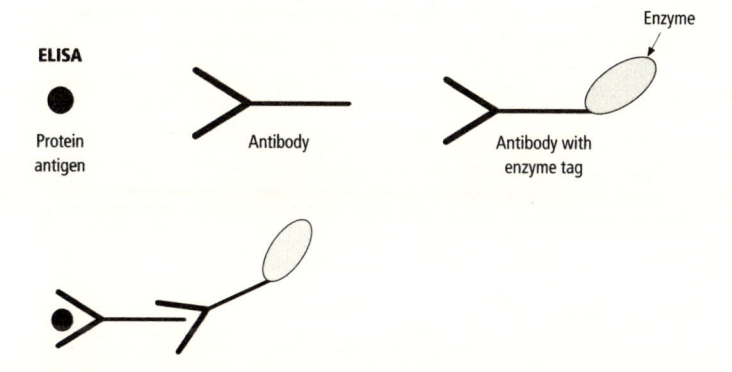

**Figure 5** Diagnostic methods. ELISA. In an ELISA, an antibody specific for the protein is used to identify the protein and then a second antibody is used to label the first antibody. This second antibody usually carries an enzymatic tag such as horseradish peroxidase which causes a colour change when appropriate chemicals are added.

## Answers • Gastroenterology

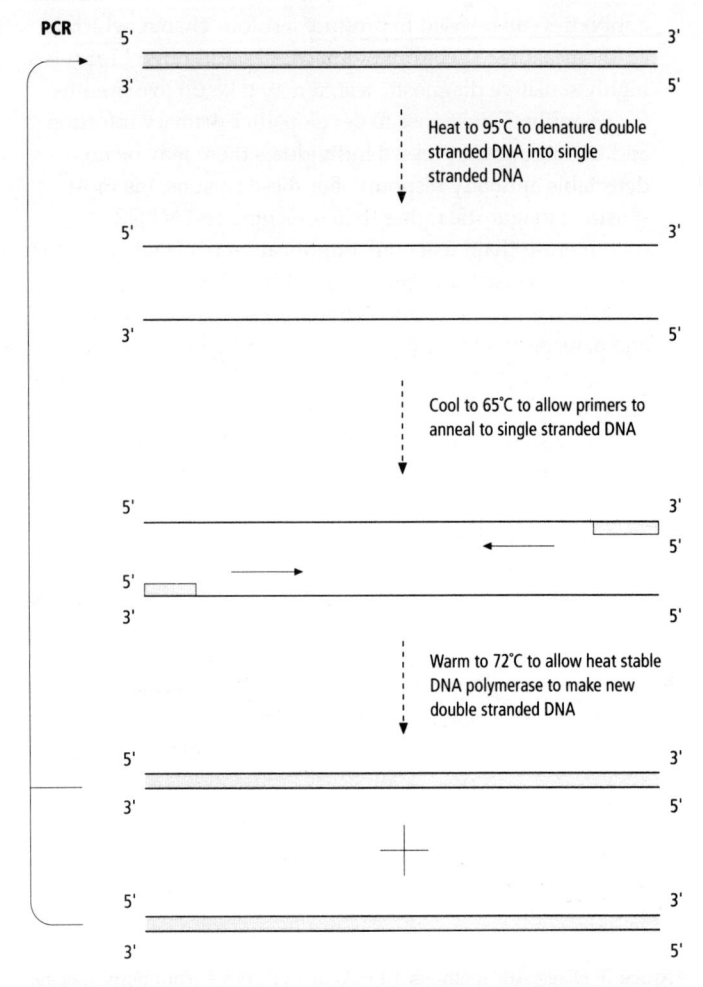

**Figure 6** Diagnostic methods. PCR. In the polymerase chain reaction (PCR), a thermostable DNA polymerase is used to amplify small quantities of DNA. Two oligonucleotide primers are used to prime transcription and the segment of DNA between them will be amplified if it is present in the material being tested.

- cigarette smoking;
- a history of peptic ulcer disease.

Of the drugs studied, ibuprofen does seem to have a low risk of gastrointestinal adverse effects compared to other NSAIDs. In Zollinger–Ellison syndrome there is overproduction of gastrin by G cells, often in the pancreas and consequent acid hypersecretion; ulcers frequently occur in the absence of *H. pylori*.

## 7 T,T,T,T,T

In Zollinger–Ellison syndrome overproduction of gastrin by G cells produces hyper-secretion of acid in the stomach. This lowers the pH in the upper jejunum which can result in diarrhoea. Hypogammaglobulinaemia is associated with gut infections which can cause diarrhoea, such as giardiasis with consequent malabsorption. Lactulose is normally broken down by colonic bacteria, but if there is bacterial overgrowth in the small intestine, the early breakdown causes an early peak in breath hydrogen. Bacterial overgrowth causes deconjugation of bile salts with resultant diarrhoea. Chronic pancreatitis with exocrine insufficiency and Whipple's disease with abnormal bowel can both cause malabsorption with accompanying steatorrhoea and diarrhoea.

## 8 T,T,F,T,T

The aetiology of irritable bowel syndrome (IBS) is unclear; psychological factors are important but it is possible that altered bowel motility or sensation play a role. Two thirds of patients are symptom free by 5 years. Investigations such as the erythrocytes sedimentation rate are usually normal. Both lactose intolerance and IBS are common and may cause similar symptoms in patients with both conditions. As the prognosis is good the key aspect of management is the exclusion of diseases which require more aggressive therapy such as neoplasia or inflammatory bowel disease.

**Answers** • Gastroenterology

### 9 T,F,T,T,F

The key forms of chronic liver disease are chronic persistent hepatitis, chronic active hepatitis and cirrhosis. The main causes of chronic active hepatitis are the hepatitis B and C viruses. Ursodeoxycholic acid (ursodiol), a bile acid, retards the progression of liver dysfunction in primary biliary cirrhosis and reduces the requirement for transplantation. Propranolol is a beta blocker and is of benefit in preventing recurrent bleeding from oesophageal varices, possibly by reducing portal hypertension. It does not alter mortality.

### 10 F,T,T,T,F

Chronic active hepatitis and cirrhosis are associated with normal or small liver size. The key diagnoses to consider with ascites and a large liver are Budd–Chiari syndrome, constrictive pericarditis and hepatocellular carcinoma or other malignancy. Budd–Chiari syndrome occurs when there is portal vein obstruction, usually due to thrombosis. If there is a history of chronic liver disease, then a large liver should prompt a search for hepatocellular carcinoma (hepatoma) and if necessary the exclusion of portal vein thrombosis.

### 11 F,T,T,F,T

Fever occurs in both conditions. The arthropathy of ulcerative colitis invariably responds to resection of the affected bowel, but that of Crohn's disease commonly does not. The elemental diet certainly works in Crohn's disease, but its role in ulcerative colitis is not clear.

• Histologically, Crohn's disease is characterized by a lymphocytic infiltrate, granuloma formation, transmural disease and normal gland and goblet cell architecture.

• Ulcerative colitis is characterized by a polymorphonuclear infiltrate, no granulomas, distortion of the gland architecture and goblet cell depletion.

Gastroenterology • **Answers**

- In ulcerative colitis, the lesions do not normally extend throughout the full thickness of the bowel wall, whereas in Crohn's they may do so resulting in fistulas.

## 12 T,T,T,F,T

Small bowel ulcers particularly occur with slow release nonsteroidal anti-inflammatory drugs and can heal with stricture formation. Behçet's disease can cause oral, genital and ileal ulcers. Cryoglobulins are antibodies, usually anti-IgG rheumatoid factors, which precipitate at temperatures below 37°C. Cryoglobulinaemia is a well recognized association of hepatitis C virus infection. Whipple's disease is associated with infection with the extracellular bacterium *Tropheryma whippelii*, and can be treated with antibiotic combinations such as penicillin, streptomycin and cotrimoxazole (trimethoprim and sulphamethoxazole). The mechanism of partial villous atrophy in HIV infection is unclear.

## 13 T,T,F,T,T

Reactive arthritis can occur after any infection, but is often triggered by campylobacter or yersinia infection. Cryptosporidium causes a diarrhoeal illness that is usually self-limiting and does not require treatment. However, in the immunocompromised treatment may be necessary. In schistosomiasis (bilharzia), the trematodes or flukes can live in the mesenteric veins where they produce eggs. Especially if the worm burden is high, these eggs can produce a granulomatous hepatitis with subsequent periportal fibrosis and portal hypertension. This occurs with *Schistosoma mansoni* and *japonica*. With *Schistosoma haematobium* infection, the worms live in the pelvic veins and the damage occurs to the urinary tract which can result in urinary obstruction and bladder cancer. Giardiasis is caused by infection with the

## Answers • Gastroenterology

flagellate *Giardia lamblia* and like other infections can cause enterocyte damage which may result in malabsorption until it recovers.

### 14 F,T,T,T,T

The carcinoid syndrome occurs when carcinoid tumour cells release vasoactive substances which can cause flushing, tachycardia, diarrhoea and sometimes hypotension. The tumour is usually in the gut, but can also occur in the lung. With gut tumours, the syndrome only occurs when there are hepatic metastases as prior to metastasis the liver degrades many of the vasoactive compounds produced by the tumour. Many different compounds may be produced and serotonin or 5-hydroxytryptamine accounts for only some of the effects on the patient. Urinary levels of a serotonin metabolite 5-hydroxyindoleacetic acid (5-HIAA) are usually raised, but walnuts, bananas and avocados also cause raised urinary 5-HIAA levels. Tricuspid and pulmonary stenosis can occur. Octreotide is a synthetic analogue of somatostatin which is an inhibitor of many endocrine and exocrine functions and is of benefit. Nuclear scans employ labelled octreotide to highlight affected regions.

### 15 T,F,F,F,F

Primary sclerosing cholangitis is a condition with fibrosis of the entire biliary system. 75% of patients with primary sclerosing cholangitis have ulcerative colitis. 70% of patients are men. Antimitochondrial antibodies are usually negative and the best way of making the diagnosis is by ERCP (endoscopic retrograde cholangio-pancreatogram). Ursodeoxycholic acid is of proven benefit in primary biliary cirrhosis. Antimitochondrial antibodies are often positive in primary biliary cirrhosis.

## 16 T,T,T,T,F

In achalasia there is dilatation of an aperistaltic section of the oesophagus above a narrowed distal end where there is a failure of the normal relaxation of the lower oesophageal sphincter on swallowing. In systemic sclerosis there is fibrosis of the oesophagus and in diabetes an autonomic neuropathy can affect oesophageal motility. With chronic Chagas' disease mega-oesophagus can occur. Cystic fibrosis can result in chronic liver disease with oesophageal varices, but dysphagia is not a feature.

## 17 T,F,T,T,F

Persistent acid reflux can affect the chest by causing repeated aspiration with recurrent infection or by causing a worsening of asthma. There is not usually any associated acid base disorder. Persistent reflux is associated with transition of cells in the lower oesophagus to a gastric columnar epithelium (Barrett's oesophagus) which can undergo dysplastic or adenocarcinomatous change.

## 18 T,T,T,T,T

In chronic ulcer disease scarring can result in pyloric stenosis with a tendency to vomiting and concomitant bronchial aspiration of gastric contents. There is loss of $H^+$ and $Cl^-$ in the vomit with a consequent hypochloraemic alkalosis. Renal compensation for this may be inefficient with inappropriately acid urine. The reasons for this are complex. Dehydration can reduce glomerular filtration rate. $Na^+$ and $Cl^-$ are reabsorbed together from the renal tubules. Because of the low serum $Cl^-$ level there is reduced filtration of $Cl^-$ and so reduced tubular $Cl^-$ concentration and so less efficient $Na^+$ reabsorption This means that there is more tubular $Na^+$ available for $Na^+/H^+$ exchange, so there is more $H^+$ secretion. In the same way, there is more $Na^+/K^+$ exchange. In addition, the renal $H^+$ and

## Answers • Gastroenterology

K⁺ transport shares the same pump system and if there is a deficiency of H⁺ then the kidney will secrete K⁺ so producing hypokalaemia.

### 19 T,T,T,T,F

Hypoglycaemia in acute liver failure results from loss of the ability of the liver to regulate and maintain normal glucose levels. In cerebral oedema due to acute liver failure, mannitol, barbiturates, hyperventilation and upright positioning may be of benefit. Lactulose reduces bowel transit time and may reduce the load of encephalopathic substances reaching the systemic circulation from the gut in the absence of an efficient liver detoxification system. In severe encephalopathy, liver transplantation is of great benefit.

### 20 T,T,F,F,F

The commonest causes of chronic liver disease are alcohol and infection with hepatitis B or C viruses. Liver disease in cystic fibrosis is thought to result from blockage of the small bile ducts by viscid secretions. Alkaptonuria is caused by a deficiency of homogentisic acid oxidase which converts homogentisic acid to maleylacetoacetic acid. The excess homogentisic acid polymerizes and is deposited as a brown–black pigment in cartilage and fibrous tissue and can cause arthritis, but does not cause liver disease. Bartter's syndrome consists principally of hypokalaemic alkalosis with raised levels of renin, angiotensin II and aldosterone.

The porphyrias are disorders of haem synthesis and can be divided into the hepatic porphyrias in which porphyrins accumulate in the liver and the erythropoietic porphyrias in which porphyrins accumulate in red cells. The metabolic pathway of haem synthesis is shown in Fig. 7.

*Hepatic porphyrias*
Acute porphyrias
   Acute intermittent porphyria (AIP)
   Hereditary coproporphyria (HCP)
   Variegate porphyria (VP)
Nonacute porphyrias
Porphyria cutanea tarda

*Erythropoietic porphyrias*
Congenital erythropoietic porphyria
Protoporphyria

The acute porphyrias are dominantly transmitted and are characterized by a tendency to acute attacks of abdominal pain, hypertension and neuropsychiatric disturbances including peripheral neuropathies. The attacks can be triggered by infection, alcohol, sex hormones and drugs.

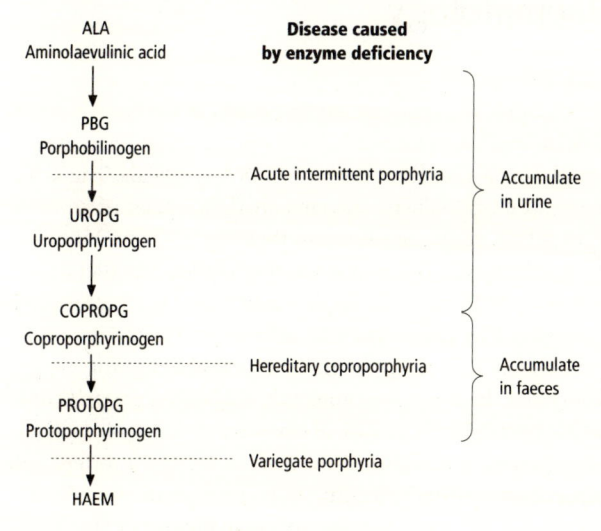

```
ALA                        Disease caused
Aminolaevulinic acid       by enzyme deficiency
     │
     ▼
   PBG
Porphobilinogen
     ┊  ············ Acute intermittent porphyria  ┐
     ▼                                              │ Accumulate
  UROPG                                             │ in urine
Uroporphyrinogen                                    │
     │                                              │
     ▼                                              │
 COPROPG                                            │
Coproporphyrinogen                                  │
     ┊  ············ Hereditary coproporphyria     ┤ Accumulate
     ▼                                              │ in faeces
 PROTOPG                                            │
Protoporphyrinogen                                  │
     ┊  ············ Variegate porphyria           ┘
     ▼
   HAEM
```

**Figure 7** Haem synthesis and the acute porphyrias.

Drugs that are particularly problematic include barbiturates, anticonvulsants, oestrogens, sulphonamides and tetracycline. Drugs generally thought to be safe include aspirin, penicillins, opiates and aminoglycosides. During an acute attack there is increased production of the metabolites preceding the site of the block. In the simplest terms the acute porphyrias can be distinguished on the following basis:
- acute intermittent porphyria-urinary porphyrins elevated;
- hereditary coproporphyria-faecal porphyrins elevated;
- variegate porphyria-urinary and faecal porphyrins elevated.

Liver disease principally occurs in congenital erythropoietic porphyria and porphyria cutanea tarda. Urinary porphyrins can be elevated in lead poisoning

# Haematology

## 1 T,T,T,T,T

In megaloblastic anaemia, erythroblasts in the bone marrow have delayed development of the nucleus relative to the cytoplasm as a result of defective DNA synthesis. The key causes of megaloblastic anaemia are deficiencies of vitamin $B_{12}$ or folate, or abnormalities of their metabolism. Vitamin $B_{12}$ deficiency can occur as a result of inadequate diet or a deficiency in intrinsic factor. Intrinsic factor is a glycoprotein synthesized by gastric parietal cells which binds vitamin $B_{12}$ and delivers it to receptors in the terminal ileum for absorption. In pernicious anaemia, antibodies are present to gastric parietal cells in 90% of cases and to intrinsic factor in 50% of cases. Antibodies to intrinsic factor can interfere with its function by direct blocking or by precipitation. Coeliac disease can reduce folate absorption in the upper small intestine. Alcohol abuse is commonly associated with folate deficiency, probably because of dietary insufficiency. Phenytoin interferes with folate metabolism, but the exact mechanism of this effect is not clear. Pregnancy results in increased folate requirements and deficiency during pregnancy is common worldwide.

## 2 T,T,T,F,F

Heparin can cause thrombocytopaenia by promoting platelet destruction. Haemolytic uraemic syndrome is principally a disease of children with gastrointestinal symptoms, acute renal failure, intravascular haemolysis and often thrombo-cytopaenia. The antiphospholipid antibody syndrome comprises thrombocytopaenia, spontaneous abortion, thrombosis and in some cases neurological changes; the syndrome can be associated with systemic lupus erythematosus. von Willebrand factor normally promotes platelet aggregation and serves as a carrier for factor VIII. In von Willebrand's disease there is a deficiency of von Willebrand factor resulting in impaired platelet function and so prolonged bleeding time, but not thrombocytopaenia.

## 3 F,T,F,T,F

There are a number of very well recognized drug interactions with warfarin.
- Drugs such as cimetidine and isoniazid inhibit the metabolic degradation of warfarin and so increases its effect.
- Phenytoin, carbamazepine, rifampicin and barbiturates such as thiopentone increase the metabolic degradation of warfarin and so reduce its effect.
- Warfarin is highly albumin bound and salicylates, phenylbutazone and sulphonamides can displace it from albumin, thereby increasing serum levels of the unbound drug and increasing its effect.

## Answers • Haematology

### 4 T,T,T,T,T

Sickle-cell disease is caused by a homozygous state for a mutation causing a substitution of valine for glutamic acid at position 6 in the beta chain of haemoglobin. The result of this is that when it becomes deoxygenated the abnormal or sickle haemoglobin forms a liquid crystal structure which ultimately results in sickling of the erythrocyte with vessel occlusion and tissue infarction. Sickle-cell trait occurs in heterozygotes for the mutation and under these circumstances, sickling only occurs with severe hypoxia, as for example, a complication of anaesthesia. In children, dactylitis, a painful swelling of the hands and feet can be the first presentation. Hyposplenism can occur as the spleen is damaged by repeated infarction. This may contribute to an increased susceptibility to infection. Particularly in tropical countries, salmonella osteomyelitis can occur. Sickle-cell disease can result in ischaemic damage to the kidneys, mesangiocapillary glomerulonephritis and proteinuria. A sickle cell crisis affecting the lung can cause hypoxia. It is noteworthy that heterozygotes seem relatively resistant to severe falciparum malaria.

### 5 T,T,T,F,F

In beta-thalassaemia major both beta-globin genes are abnormal and the excess normal alpha chains precipitate in the red cell precursors causing ineffective erythropoeisis and haemolysis. Extramedullary (that is outside the bone marrow) erythropoeisis occurs with enlargement of the liver and spleen. In beta-thalassaemia trait there is usually an abnormality of one beta-globin gene, which may result in a hypochromic microcytic blood picture with or without a degree of anaemia. If two people with beta-thalassaemia trait have a child, there is a 1 in 4 chance of beta-thalassaemia major occurring. Chronic infection with schistosomes can

Haematology • **Answers**

cause hepatic inflammation with granuloma formation and portal fibrosis resulting in portal hypertension, with a consequently large liver and spleen. Visceral leishmaniasis can occur with parasite multiplication in the spleen and sometimes liver and consequent enlargement of these organs. Aplastic anaemia results from a failure of haemopoeitic stem cell proliferation and the liver and spleen are not enlarged.

## 6 T,F,F,T,F

In paroxysmal nocturnal haemoglobinuria, there is excessive sensitivity to the lytic effects of complement on red cells and to some extent on white cells and platelets. Red cell lysis is easily demonstrated at low pH (acid lysis or Ham's test).

- Cryoglobulins are usually anti-IgG antibodies ('rheumatoid factors') which precipitate at temperatures below 37°C
- Cold agglutinins are antibodies which cause greater agglutination of red blood cells at 4°C than at 37°C. Mycoplasma infection is often associated with polyclonal IgM cold agglutinins which may be responsible for haemolysis as they are directed against the I antigen on erythrocytes.

In thiamine deficiency, red cell transketolase activity is reduced, but returns to normal after addition of the cofactor thiamine pyrophosphate. Granulocytes produce the serum vitamin $B_{12}$ binding protein transcobalamin 1 and this is increased in chronic granulocytic leukaemia with a consequent rise in serum vitamin $B_{12}$. The Philadelphia chromosome is a translocation arising between chromosome 9 and chromosome 22 and is found in 95% of patients with chronic granulocytic leukaemia. This translocation places the cellular proto-oncogene c-*abl* close to the breakpoint cluster region (*bcr*) on chromosome 22 and results in active transcription of an altered form of c-*abl* which is a protein kinase and may be involved in leukaemogenesis.

**Answers** • Haematology

### 7 T,T,F,T,T

Haemoglobin is a tetramer of two alpha and two beta chains which contain haem molecules and reversibly bind oxygen. Binding of oxygen by one chain increases the affinity of the others and this co-operativity means that the dissociation curve is sigmoid shaped. Oxygen affinity is decreased by increasing carbon dioxide concentrations, a fall in pH or a rise in 2,3-diphosphoglycerate (2,3-DPG). Any mutation interfering with the production of efficient haemoglobin may contribute to thalassaemia and mutations in noncoding introns or in the upstream promoter regions of the globin genes are known to do this. There are two main beta-globin genes on chromosome 11 and four main alpha-globin genes on chromosome 16, respectively.

### 8 F,F,T,F,F

The peak incidence of acute myeloid leukaemia is in adult life, whereas acute lymphoblastic leukaemia has a peak in childhood and a better prognosis with treatment. Most cases of acute myeloid leukaemia will arise as a result of uncontrolled proliferation of an abnormal blast cell and subsequent replacement of normal bone marrow cells by leukaemia cells. The syndrome of bone marrow failure can then occur with anaemia, leucopaenia and thrombocytopaenia. In normal cells destined to become T cells, the T-cell receptor genes undergo a rearrangement process to produce a functional T-cell receptor.
• In acute myeloid leukaemia, the blasts usually show some evidence of differentiation towards the granulocyte lines and T-cell receptor genes are not normally rearranged.
• However, in acute lymphoblastic leukaemia there may be early lymphoid differentiation and this may be detected by rearrangement of immunoglobulin or T-cell receptor genes.

In acute myeloid leukaemia, but not acute lymphoblastic leukaemia, Sudan black and myeloperoxidase staining may

Haematology • **Answers**

be positive. Renal failure is a rare complication resulting from direct infiltration of the kidneys, urate nephropathy secondary to cell lysis or sepsis. Nephrotic syndrome is not characteristic of the disease.

## 9 T,T,F,F,T

The peak incidence of chronic granulocytic leukaemia is between 50 and 60 years with a median survival of around 3–4 years and in about 70% of patients a transformation to acute leukaemia will occur. Massive splenomegaly often with some hepatomegaly is common. The peripheral white cell count is high, but there may be anaemia and thrombocytopaenia. Chemotherapy can reduce tumour bulk and help symptoms, but only bone marrow transplantation is curative and this is usually only carried out in young and fit patients.

## 10 T,T,T,T,T

There are many causes of a tendency to thrombosis including deficiencies of protein C, protein S or antithrombin III, resistance to protein C and the presence of an anticardiolipin antibody with lupus anticoagulant activity. Antithrombin III modulates the procoagulant activity of thrombin. Thrombin binds to thrombomodulin on the endothelial cell and by doing this becomes an anticoagulant protein which activates the serine protease protein C. Protein C inactivates factors VIIIa and Va in the presence of its cofactor protein S. Factor V Leiden is a mutation in factor V which renders it resistant to cleavage by protein C. In nephrotic syndrome there may be loss of regulatory proteins in the urine. The lupus anticoagulant is an antibody to phospholipids which interferes with the binding of phospholipid to form prothrombin activator and causes a prolonged activated partial thromboplastin time (APPT) and a paradoxical tendency to thrombosis.

**Answers** • Haematology

## 11 T,T,T,T,T

The key causes of a microcytic blood picture are:
- iron deficiency;
- thalassaemia;
- sideroblastic anaemia.

Iron deficiency usually results from blood loss, usually menstrual or gastrointestinal in the UK. In countries where parasitic worms are prevalent, anaemia frequently results from gastrointestinal loss due to hookworm infestation. The characteristic changes with iron deficiency are a reduction in serum iron and serum ferritin and an increase in serum total iron binding capacity. Serum ferritin represents iron storage and total iron binding capacity may reflect an increased effort to absorb iron from the gut. However, ferritin is an acute phase protein and can therefore be elevated even in the presence of iron deficiency if there is generalized inflammation. A good check on this if there is doubt is to measure the C reactive protein (CRP) at the same time. If the CRP, which is also an acute phase marker, is normal then the ferritin is probably a good index of iron storage. Sideroblastic anaemia results from an inherited or acquired defect in haem synthesis and can result in microcytosis or macrocytosis.

## 12 T,T,T,T,T

Glucose-6-phosphate dehydrogenase deficiency (G-6-PD) is an X-linked disorder in which the low enzyme level predisposes the red cells to haemolysis in the presence of oxidant drugs. The key drug groups causing this are:
- the aminoquinolines such as chloroquine and primaquine;
- the sulphones such as dapsone;
- the sulphonamides;
- the nitrofurans;
- the aspirin-like analgesics.

Haematology • **Answers**

## 13 T,T,F,T,T

Myeloma is a plasma cell neoplasm, associated with secretion of a paraprotein. Typical features include lytic bone lesions, hypercalcaemia, renal impairment, bleeding, infection, hyperviscosity syndrome and sometimes amyloidosis. The key prognostic indicators in the Medical Research Council myeloma trials have been serum urea, haemoglobin and clinical disability (*British Journal of Cancer* 1980: **42**; 831–40). There may be reduced levels of normal immunoglobulins and defective antibody responses. The production of osteoclast activating factor (OAF) contributes to the typical multiple skeletal erosions by promoting bone destruction by osteoclasts.

## 14 T,T,T,T,T

The hyperviscosity syndrome occurs when the viscosity of blood is sufficient to impair microcirculatory flow. This may occur with high levels of paraproteins, especially IgM. Clinical features include headache, drowsiness, haemorrhage, neuropathy, retinopathy and cardiac failure. Plasmapheresis removes plasma containing the paraprotein and can rapidly improve the symptoms.

## 15 T,T,T,F,T

The main vitamin K-dependent clotting factors are II, VII, IX and X. Haemophilia prolongs the activated partial thromboplastin time (APTT). von Willebrand's disease results from a deficiency of von Willebrand factor which normally promotes platelet aggregation and serves as a carrier for factor VIII; bleeding time is prolonged because of impaired platelet function. Plasmin promotes clot lysis by the conversion of fibrin to fibrin degradation products, hence the use of plasminogen activators to convert plasminogen to plasmin in thrombolysis. Thrombin promotes the conversion of fibrinogen to fibrin during clot formation. Platelet function is impaired in chronic renal failure resulting in a prolonged bleeding time.

## 16 F,T,T,F,T

In the foetus, B cells develop in the liver, whereas in adults the bone marrow is the site of B cell production. Interleukin-6 plays a key role in inducing B cells to differentiate into antibody producing plasma cells and is thought to be important as a growth factor for myeloma. During T cell development in the thymus there appears to be significant death of T cell precursors by apoptosis (programmed cell death). T cell precursors that are auto-reactive are deleted and T cells that may recognize foreign antigenic peptide bound to self major histocompatibility complex antigen are selected for further development. Circulating monocytes can become tissue macrophages. Granulocyte-macrophage colony stimulating factor (GM–CSF) increases the production of neutrophils and monocytes and can be of use in reducing the duration of neutropaenia during cancer chemotherapy. Eosinophils, neutrophils and basophils are all granulocytes.

## 17 T,T,T,T,T

In rheumatoid arthritis anaemia can be the result of chronic inflammatory disease itself, gastrointestinal bleeding secondary to nonsteroidal anti-inflammatory drugs or bone marrow suppression from drugs, such as azathioprine. Any cause of chronic renal failure can result in anaemia because of erythropoietin deficiency. Around 10–15% of patients with chronic lymphocytic leukaemia develop an auto-immune haemolytic anaemia with a positive direct Coomb's test. In the more severe forms of Ehlers–Danlos syndrome, there is a bleeding tendency, with rupture of small vessels which are inadequately supported because of defective collagen synthesis.

## 18 T,F,F,F,T

Coeliac disease is associated with an increased incidence of small bowel lymphomas. In Hodgkin's disease fever, weight loss and night sweats are known as B symptoms. Although the prognosis of high grade non-Hodgkin's lymphoma is worse than that of low grade disease, low grade disease is not usually curable, whereas a number of patients with high grade disease do seem to achieve a long-term cure.

- Mycosis fungoides is a scaly skin lesion of lymphoma type with a good prognosis.
- Sézary syndrome is a red, eczematous and sometimes pigmented skin lymphoma with a worse prognosis.

## 19 T,T,T,T,F

Promyelocytic leukaemia accounts for about 10% of all cases of acute myeloid leukaemia. Presentation is often with a bleeding diathesis. Malignant promyelocytes release procoagulant substances that activate the clotting cascade and can cause depletion of clotting factors and fibrinogen. Typically there is a balanced and reciprocal translocation between the long arms of chromosomes 15 and 17 which is associated with rearrangement of the retinoic acid receptor alpha ($RAR\alpha$) gene, placing it next to a gene called *PML* and resulting in a fusion gene coding for a new transcript. Retinoids are derived from vitamin A and are involved in regulating cell differentiation. Tretinoin (all trans retinoic acid) causes differentiation of immature neoplastic cells into mature granulocytes and so promotes remission.

## 20 T,F,T,T,F

Antibodies to the A and B antigens commonly occur in the absence of previous exposure to blood. These 'naturally occurring' antibodies may result from exposure to bacteria displaying similar antigens. The commonest antibody arising

## Answers • Haematology/Infection

from sensitization is directed against the D antigen of the Rhesus system. If a mother is Rhesus negative, her foetus can inherit the Rhesus antigen from the father and be Rhesus positive. During the pregnancy or birth, the mother may be exposed and sensitized to foetal Rhesus antigens and this can cause problems during blood transfusion or subsequent pregnancy. Anti-Rhesus immunoglobulin given perinatally reduces the chance of the mother becoming immunized by promoting the destruction and removal of any foetal red cells from the maternal circulation. Antibodies to ABO incompatible blood cause complement activation and red cell lysis. Complement components, such as C3a, C4a and C5a, contribute to symptoms and hypotension. Reactions to white cell antigens usually cause febrile reactions. Pulmonary infiltrates can occur if the donor plasma contains antibodies which agglutinate the recipients granulocytes. Radiographic infiltrates can sometimes be seen with fever, cough and dyspnoea. In a crossmatch, an indirect Coomb's test is performed by exposing donor cells to recipient serum and then adding antihuman immunoglobulin. In a positive crossmatch, antibodies to the donor cell are present in the recipient serum and bind the cells; when antihuman globulin is added visual red cell agglutination occurs.

# Infection

### 1 F,F,T,T,T

*Clostridium tetani* is a Gram-positive spore forming rod, which lives principally in soil. Immunization is with tetanus toxoid, an inactivated form of tetanus toxin. Tetanus toxin is also called tetanospasmin and acts especially at presynaptic sites on inhibitory cells in the motor system. A central result is a blockade of the gamma-amino-butyric acid (GABA) pathway in the motor system. Blockade of this inhibitory system results in instability and overactivity of the motor system and so muscle spasm. Dysphagia can be an early symptom. Late in the disease, autonomic instability with fluctuating heart rates and blood pressure can occur. Benzodiazepines can relieve the spasm which can make artificial ventilation easier if it is required. Although penicillin is of benefit, metronidazole is the preferred drug.

## 2 F,F,T,T,T

Leprosy is caused by *Mycobacterium leprae* and bacille Calmette–Guérin (BCG) vaccination in trials in Malawi and Venezuela has produced a protective efficacy of just over 50% (*Lancet* 1996; **348**: 17–24; *Lancet* 1992; **339**: 446–50). The disease is a clinical spectrum with the two ends defined by tuberculoid and lepromatous disease. Many patients display a clinical picture which does not fall discretely into one of these categories.

- Tuberculoid leprosy is localized within an area of hypopigmented, anaesthetic skin. The local peripheral nerves may be thickened and recovery can occur spontaneously. Cellular immunity is intact and active with T helper 1 cells (TH1) producing interleukin-2 (IL-2) and interferon gamma.
- Lepromatous leprosy is a more advanced stage of disease and is generalized. Cellular immunity to the organism is functionally less active with T helper 2 cells (TH2) predominating. These cells typically secrete interleukins 4, 5 and 10. There may be infiltration of tissues resulting in macules, papules or nodules and thickening of tissues such as the ear lobes. Tissue destruction can ultimately occur.

## 3 T,T,T,T,T

Lyme disease is caused by the spirochaete *Borrelia burgdorferi* and is carried by the hard bodied ixodid ticks which have a worldwide distribution.

## Answers • Infection

- Usually the only manifestation is a rash known as erythema chronicum migrans which spreads out from the tickbite with a red migrating edge.
- In the later stages, potential targets include the skin, central nervous system, heart and joints.

Nerve palsies may occur and the cerebrospinal fluid can show a lymphocytosis and slightly raised protein. A mild meningitis or peripheral neuropathy can occur. Carditis can affect the heart and myalgia and recurrent arthralgia or arthritis are well recognized. Diagnosis is usually by detection of specific antibodies in the serum, but detection of the DNA from the organism by the polymerase chain reaction is increasingly useful. Treatment is with penicillins such as amoxycillin or benzyl penicillin. Doxycycline and cephalosporins such as cefotaxime can be used if penicillin is contra-indicated because of allergy.

### 4 T,F,T,T,T

The main form of malaria prophylaxis remains the avoidance of mosquito bites. Chloroquine resistance is present in most sub-Saharan countries. If chloroquine resistance is suspected in a patient with malaria, quinine is currently the drug of choice. Mefloquine resistance does occur in the Far East, including Thailand and Cambodia.

- Chloroquine is a relatively safe drug, though retinal toxicity can occur over prolonged periods of use with a total dose of over 100g.
- Mefloquine has been associated with neuropsychiatric side-effects such as depression, anxiety, sleep disturbances and convulsions.
- Halofantrine can prolong the QT interval on the electrocardiogram, particularly when used to treat patients who have been taking mefloquine prophylaxis.

## 5 F,T,T,T,F

Toxacara is a worm which is usually transmitted to man through the faeces of dogs. Two clinical syndromes exist; ocular toxocariasis and visceral larva migrans. In the first case, granulomas occur in the eye and may interfere with vision. In visceral larva migrans, there may be gross organomegaly with fever, eosinophilia and cough or asthma. Treatment is with diethylcarbamazine or thiabendazole, but is not always satisfactory.

## 6 F,F,T,T,T

The sandfly *Phlebotomus* is the vector for the parasite which in visceral leishmaniasis is *Leishmania donovani*. In cutaneous leishmaniasis, there are a number of different *Leishmania* which can cause disease and are prevalent in different regions of the world. The tetse fly is a vector for trypanosomiasis. The two recognized types of disease are cutaneous and visceral leishmaniasis.

- In cutaneous leishmaniasis, the disease is localized to the skin with crusted or ulcerated lesions. The response to injection of dead parasites is known as the Leishmania test and it is positive in cutaneous leishmaniasis.
- Visceral leishmaniasis (kala azar) occurs late with fever, hepatosplenomegaly and impaired immunity despite raised immunoglobulin levels. Infection is common and the Leishmania test is negative.

The mainstay of treatment is with pentavalent antimonial drugs, but resistance does occur and amphotericin, particularly in liposomal preparations has proved useful.

## 7 T,T,T,T,T

The retrovirus infects CD4+ T cells by binding of the viral surface antigen gp120 to the CD4 molecule. The virus may also use recently identified chemokine receptors CXCR4 and CCR5 on the cell surface as co-receptors to enter target cells during infection and it appears that polymorphisms or deletions in the chemokine receptors may influence patient survival. There is a progressive loss of CD4+ T cells with a growing tendency to infection with other organisms. The virus also enters neural cells and many different neurological pictures can result including severe dementia. *Cryptococcus* typically causes a meningitis and cryptosporidium causes diarrhoea. Infection with mycobacterium tuberculosis and with atypical mycobacteria, such as *kansasii*, is a major problem.

## 8 T,T,T,T,T

Schistosomiasis is caused by flatworms which have their asexual phase in freshwater snails. The worms enter the skin and live in the venous system of affected organs. Acute disease can cause an itch initially, then at about 1–2 months fever and malaise can occur, sometimes with diarrhoea. Chronic disease results from the large worm burden and the allergic response to the worm eggs.

• *Schistosomiasis mansoni* and *japonicum* principally affect the gut and liver and can result in portal hypertension

• *Schistosomiasis haematobium* principally affects the urinary tract and can result in urinary tract obstruction and cancer.

Involvement of the liver causes portal hypertension, though liver function is often well preserved. Pulmonary infection can cause pulmonary hypertension and cor pulmonale. Treatment is with praziquantel.

## 9 T,T,T,F,T

Influenza virus is an RNA orthomyxovirus. The typical clinical syndrome including fever, myalgia and

nasopharyngeal symptoms is well known and can be complicated by secondary bacterial infection in the chest.
- Antigenic shift occurs through major genetic recombination of the genes for haemagglutinin or neuraminidase.
- Antigenic drift occurs by small mutations in these genes.

The vaccine is not live and can safely be used in pregnancy. The vaccine is however, grown in hens eggs prior to formalin inactivation and so cannot be given to those allergic to egg. Amantadine and rimantadine offer some protection against influenza A, but not influenza B.

## 10 T,T,T,T,T

Many viral infections can cause a hepatitis, but this is especially so with the hepatitis viruses themselves and with the herpes viruses – Epstein–Barr virus, cytomegalovirus and varicella zoster virus. Many other infections can cause jaundice including malaria. The mechanism of infection associated jaundice may be either haemolysis or impaired liver function.

## 11 T,F,T,T,F

The Chlamydiae are obligate intracellular bacteria. They are divided into two species, *Chlamydia trachomatis* and *Chlamydia psittaci*.
- *C. psittaci* causes psittacosis, an atypical pneumonia which may be transmitted from animals, especially birds.
- *C. trachomatis* causes a chronic follicular conjunctivitis which causes corneal scarring and can result in blindness. Genital infections with *C. trachomatis* include urethritis, cervicitis and lymphogranuloma venereum.

Lymphogranuloma venereum can result in painful inguinal lymphadenopathy, systemic malaise, a haemorrhagic proctitis and, rarely, genital elephantiasis.

**Answers** • Infection

**12 T,T,T,T,T**

Falciparum malaria is a serious disease and can be associated with multiple organ failure. Acute renal failure can occur with massive haemolysis and haemoglobinuria in so-called 'blackwater fever', but can also occur without massive haemolysis. Hypoglycaemia can occur and may be a particular problem when intravenous quinine is used. Regular glucose testing is mandatory. With cerebral malaria, a range of neurological abnormalities may occur, including fits, acute confusion and coma. Secondary bacterial infection can be lethal and regular screening for this is wise.

**13 F,T,F,T,T**

*Salmonella typhi* is a Gram-negative rod and can cause typhoid fever. The combination of fever and abdominal symptoms should always raise a suspicion of typhoid fever especially in a tropical context. The organism is usually ingested from food or water and can multiply in food before ingestion. After ingestion it enters the body through the gut wall and usually multiplies in locations including the gall bladder. Secondary invasion of the bowel occurs with a vigorous inflammatory response. Perforation and bleeding can occur and there is fever. Other organs such as the kidney, liver and lungs can be affected and late abscess formation can occur. Rose spots are pink macules seen mainly on the trunk. The organism can be cultured from blood, stool or in some cases urine. The Widal test measures nonspecific antibodies to the somatic O and flagellar H antigens, but is nonspecific. Treatment is with ciprofloxacin, amoxycillin, a cephalosporin or chloramphenicol.

**14 T,T,T,T,T**

Any form of immunosuppression, such as steroid therapy or HIV infection can become a risk factor for fungal infections, the defences against which are dependent on efficient T cell activity. Broad spectrum antibiotics alter the natural flora, especially in the mouth and vagina and this facilitates growth of the fungus. In diabetes there is a generalized tendency to infection, possibly because of impaired neutrophil function by the raised sugar levels. Both pregnancy and diabetes can alter vaginal pH, so predisposing to local infection.

**15 T,T,T,F,F**

Amoebic disease is usually caused by the protozoan organism *Entamoeba histolytica* and can result in a diarrhoeal illness with blood and mucus in the stool and invasion of the bowel wall by the organism. If the infection is not eradicated, it can recur for many years. At any stage, amoeba can enter the liver via the portal vein and form an abscess, which can rupture into adjacent tissues. For this reason therapeutic drainage is often required. Metronidazole is the drug of choice for amoebic infection. Serological tests may be of use, with detectable antibodies present in most patients with amoebic dysentery and almost all with amoebic liver abscesses. The finding of cysts in the stools is also useful.

**16 T,T,T,T,T**

Infections with worms are widespread and in many cases asymptomatic. There is often a degree of eosinophilia with worm infections.

- The round worms *Ascaris lumbricoides* are long worms up to 40 cm in length which live in the intestine and can cause mechanical obstruction.
- Threadworms (*Enterobius vermicularis*) are small and relatively harmless, but can cause perianal discomfort and itch.
- The two major types of hookworm are *Necator americanus* and *Ancylostoma duodenale* and the main problem is of gastrointestinal blood loss causing chronic anaemia. The worms

## Answers • Infection

live in the small intestine and attach to the intestinal mucosa using the teeth or cutting plates in their buccal capsule which results in blood loss.

• *Strongyloides stercoralis* infection can cause a recurrent itchy urticarial rash (*Larva migrans*) along the track of worm migration through the skin. This can recur many years after the initial infection. In addition, there can be abdominal and sometimes pulmonary symptoms, depending on the worm burden.

• Whipworm infection (*Trichuris trichuria*) is usually asymptomatic but can cause diarrhoea or anaemia.

### 17 T,T,F,F,T

Multiple therapy is always used in tuberculosis to prevent the emergence of treatment resistant strains over the long treatment period.

• Isoniazid can cause a peripheral neuropathy, but this does not usually occur if pyridoxine is given simultaneously.

• Streptomycin, like gentamicin can cause impaired hearing by toxicity to the vestibulo-cochlear system.

• Ethambutol can cause a dose related optic neuritis with reduced visual acuity, and sometimes central scotoma or peripheral field defects. It is important to advise patients to report any visual changes with ethambutol and if high doses are used for long periods, ophthalmological review may be of benefit to detect any early deterioration.

• Rifampicin induces liver enzymes and can cause hepatic damage. This hepatic enzyme induction accelerates the metabolism of the contraceptive pill, so reducing its efficacy.

### 18 T,T,T,F,F

Most human streptococcal disease is caused by Group A streptococci. In contrast, Group B streptococci usually cause serious disease in neonates and only rarely in adults. Group

Infection • **Answers**

B streptococci are commensal organisms in the vagina. Staphylococcal food poisoning is rapid in onset, often occurring only a few hours after ingestion of the food due to the result of the toxin. Diphtheria is a toxin producing Gram-positive rod.

19 **F,F,T,T,F**

Hydatid disease is a result of the larvae of small animal tapeworms growing in man and can occur in the UK. The usual hosts for the disease are dogs, sheep and cattle and for this reason human infection is usually related to animal rearing. The organisms responsible are *Echinococcus granulosus* and *Echinococcus multilocularis*. In hydatid disease 70% of cysts develop in the liver, with 20% in the lungs and the rest elsewhere. The cysts may keep growing and rupture, or may stop growing and calcify. Eosinophilia is usually present. *Taenia solium* is a pig tapeworm which causes cysticercosis, a different disease characterized by cerebral lesions with variable neurological consequences including epilepsy.

20 **T,T,F,T,T**

The human immunodeficiency virus can infect CD4+ T cells. CD4+ cells are killed and their numbers fall progressively throughout the disease. The virus is an RNA virus and has a *pol* gene which encodes a reverse transcriptase; this converts viral RNA to DNA which can integrate with the host cell genome. The virus can also infect nervous tissue and so cause a range of neurological abnormalities including dementia and peripheral and autonomic neuropathies. Gancylovir is a useful agent against cytomegalovirus infection, but can cause serious bone marrow depression.

# Nephrology

**1 T,T,T,T,T**

Under normal circumstances the kidney plays a critical role in excreting potassium, phosphate and urea as well as many other substances. All these substances accumulate in renal failure. Along with this there is some inevitable excretion of sodium and water, though the kidney is well designed to conserve both these substances. Creatinine is excreted by the kidney, hence its use in estimating renal function, but is only present in micromolar quantities unlike the other substances which are present in millimolar quantities.

**2 F,T,T,F,F**

Cyclosporin is metabolized in the liver by the cytochrome P-450 containing mixed oxidases and renal impairment does not affect its metabolism. Fluconazole does have renal excretion and achieves high concentrations in the urine. Nitrofurantoin is excreted in the urine. Nifedipine and hydrallazine are excreted by the liver. If the principal means of drug elimination is by the kidney, then it us usual to reduce the dosage in renal impairment.

**3 F,F,F,T,T**

Dopamine is eliminated by metabolism, rather than renal excretion. Minoxidil and metoprolol are excreted by the liver. Cimetidine is cleared by the liver, but metabolites accumulate if the glomerular filtration rate (GFR) is less than 20 ml/min. Allopurinol is metabolized to the active metabolite oxypurinol which is retained in renal impairment. Indomethacin has significant renal excretion.

**4 T,T,T,F,F**

Nonsteroidal anti-inflammatories such as indomethacin have significant renal side-effects. Normally there is tonic

Nephrology • **Answers**

prostaglandin induced renal vasodilatation. Nonsteroidal anti-inflammatory drugs inhibit prostaglandin synthesis and so block this vasodilatation. A reduction in renal vasodilatation reduces both renal blood flow and glomerular filtration rate and if severe can produce ischaemia. Cyclosporin exerts a net renal vasoconstrictive effect by increasing renal vascular tone, especially in the afferent arterioles and so reduces glomerular filtration rate. Aminoglycosides such as gentamicin cause tubular damage, usually by a toxic effect on the renal tubular epithelium.

5 **T,F,T,T,F**

The three common organisms in community acquired urinary tract infection are *Escherichia coli*, *Proteus* and *Klebsiella* species. True candida infection in the urine is not common, though superficial genital infection is.

6 **T,T,T,F,F**

The classic combination with renal artery stenosis is of high blood pressure and impaired renal function. The condition is often bilateral and the natural history is of progressive stenosis and occlusion. The pathophysiology is illustrated in Fig. 8. When the blood supply to the kidneys is compromised by renal artery stenosis there may be a fall in renal blood flow and glomerular filtration rate. In addition to this, there is increased renin secretion by the kidney. This increases the production of angiotensin II and aldosterone. Angiotensin II and aldosterone promote vasoconstriction and salt retention and high blood pressure results. Although inhibition of the angiotensin converting enzyme with captopril would seem logical to control the blood pressure, the high levels of angiotensin II can be critical in maintaining efferent arteriolar constriction. When this constriction is removed glomerular filtration rate can fall dramatically. If both kidneys are affected, acute renal failure can result.

## Answers • Nephrology

### 7 F,F,F,T,F

Membranous nephropathy is the commonest cause of nephrotic syndrome in adults in the UK. Around 10–20% of patients may progress to end stage renal disease. Most cases are idiopathic, but around 5–10% of cases are associated with

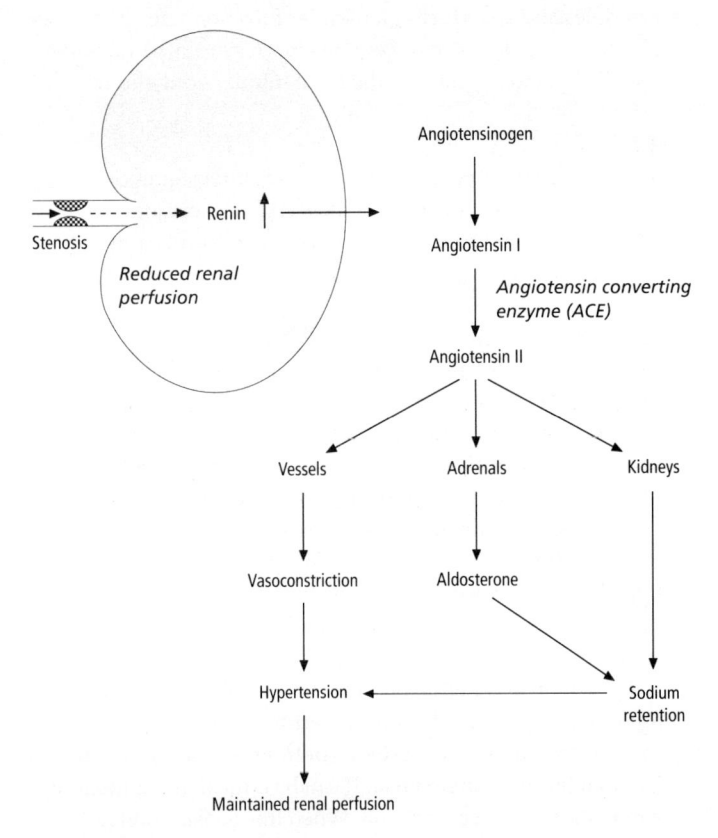

**Figure 8** Renal artery stenosis.

malignancy and a membranous nephropathy can occur in systemic lupus erythematosus, hepatitis B virus infection and with gold or penicillamine use. Spontaneous remission is usual, but some patients develop severe persistent nephrotic syndrome or progressive loss of renal function. Immunosuppression with chlorambucil and steroids (the Ponticelli regimen) has been shown to be of benefit for these patients. Frank haematuria is not a characteristic of membranous nephropathy.

## 8 T,F,T,T,F

Adrenaline is a generalized vasoconstrictor causing reduced renal blood flow. Dopamine used at the conventional dose of 1–5mcg/kg/min increases renal blood flow. For this reason, it is conventional to give dopamine when adrenaline is used to protect renal blood flow. Captopril and indomethacin can both cause a reduction in glomerular filtration rate (*see answers 4 and 6 above*). Captopril may reduce glomerular filtration rate by lowering efferent arteriolar tone.

## 9 F,T,T,T,F

Worldwide, IgA nephropathy is probably the commonest glomerulonephritis. The classic history is of recurrent frank red haematuria, often following an infective illness. Nephrotic syndrome does occur, but is not common. End stage renal failure can occur. Bad prognostic signs include male sex, hypertension and renal impairment at diagnosis. Treatment is not of any clear benefit for most patients.

## 10 F,F,F,F,F

Electron microscopy shows fusion of the epithelial foot processes or podocytes in minimal change nephropathy. There are by definition no changes on routine light microscopy or immunofluorescence – hence the name 'minimal

### Answers • Nephrology

change' nephropathy. Most patients make a full recovery when treated with steroids. In resistant cases, more aggressive immunosuppression with cyclosporin has been used successfully. Nephrotic syndrome is the normal clinical presentation. Associated features are often a recent history of infection and a history of atopy.

**11 F,T,F,F,T**

Focal segmental glomerular sclerosis is the most common cause of nephrotic syndrome in children, but accounts for only 25% of cases in adults. Some nephrologists regard minimal change disease and focal glomerular sclerosis as being essentially two ends of the same disease spectrum. In both diseases there is heavy proteinuria with foot process fusion and no significant immunoglobulin or complement deposition in the glomerulus – hence the negative immunofluorescence. However, whereas with minimal change disease a response to steroids is normal, focal segmental glomerular sclerosis is often resistant to treatment. Most patients with focal glomerulosclerosis have progressive loss of renal function and many are nephrotic. There is an association with heroin addiction. Recurrence in transplants can be rapid.

**12 F,F,F,F,F**

Almost all patients with diabetic nephropathy have retinopathy. Micro-albuminuria is the first sign and haematuria is not a characteristic feature. Angiotensin converting enzyme inhibitors may slow the rate of renal deterioration, but not diuretics. Transplantation is not contra-indicated, but is slightly less successful than in nondiabetics. Hypertension develops in almost all diabetic patients as renal function deteriorates.

Nephrology • **Answers**

## 13 T,F,F,F,F

Hypertension is extremely common and most patients do not have any underlying cause and do not develop renal damage. Proteinuria can occur, but is not usually heavy. Haematuria does not usually occur. There is good evidence that treating elevations of systolic blood pressure alone is of benefit.

## 14 T,F,T,T,T

Penicillamine and gold are recognized causes of membranous nephropathy. Although hydrallazine causes a lupus like disease, renal involvement is very rare. Acyclovir can crystallize in the urine and cause tubular damage; for this reason hydration is important when acyclovir is given systemically. Amphotericin can cause tubular and occasionally glomerular damage.

## 15 T,T,F,F,F

The nephrotic syndrome occurs when there is proteinuria sufficient to cause hypoalbuminaemia, usually with peripheral oedema. By definition serum albumin is reduced in nephrotic syndrome. As in the three oedema states, that is congestive heart failure, chronic liver failure and nephrotic syndrome there is vigorous sodium retention by the kidney resulting in fluid retention and oedema. 10% of adult nephrotics have clinically evident thrombosis at some stage. It has been suggested that this is because of urinary loss of proteins involved in the regulation of coagulation. Protein restriction results in malnourished patients and does not alter the disease process. There is often substantial hyper-lipidaemia, though the reasons for this are poorly understood.

## 16 F,F,F,F,F

Renal tubular acidosis results from a reduced ability to

excrete an acid urine and hence there is a systemic acidosis with a normal anion gap. Because there is acidaemia, serum bicarbonate is lowered and serum chloride raised. Sodium is usually normal. Potassium is usually low or normal except in type 4 renal tubular acidosis.

- In proximal renal tubular acidosis (type 2) there is reduced proximal tubular bicarbonate reabsorption, so plasma bicarbonate is low and in the acidaemic range. These patients can excrete acid when the plasma bicarbonate falls below the renal threshold at which it is fully reabsorbed. This type of renal tubular acidosis can occur alone or as part of the Fanconi syndrome in association with other tubular defects.
- In distal renal tubular acidosis (type 1) there is a defect in the secretion of hydrogen ions in the distal tubule. Unlike type 2, there is an absolute inability to secrete a maximally acid urine. Potassium and hydrogen ions share the same pump and so potassium may be substituted for hydrogen ions resulting in hypokalaemia. Urinary citrate is usually low, for reasons which are unclear and urinary calcium concentrations may be high. Causes include nephrocalcinosis, genetic disorders and autoimmune disorders such as Sjögren's syndrome.
- Type 3 renal tubular acidosis refers to patients who have features of both proximal and distal tubular acidoses.
- Type 4 renal tubular acidosis usually occurs when aldosterone levels are low. As aldosterone normally enhances renal potassium excretion, serum potassium is high and potassium is excreted in preference to hydrogen ions resulting in systemic acidaemia.

## 17 T,T,T,T,T

Nephrocalcinosis is a diffuse increase in the calcium content of the kidney substance, often causing extensive macroscopic calcification. Any long-term cause of hypercalcaemia can cause nephrocalcinosis such as hyperparathyroidism, sarcoidosis and milk alkali syndrome (which involves excessive calcium intake). Medullary sponge kidney is a congenital renal abnormality with ectatic abnormalities of the collecting system.

## 18 F,F,F,F,T,

The adult and juvenile diseases are different; the adult disease is dominant and the juvenile disease is recessive. The rate of renal deterioration is variable and only around 50% of patients have reached end stage renal disease by the age of 70. Hypertension is very common and frank haematuria is well recognized. Urinary tract infection is common. Extra renal manifestations include liver cysts and intracranial aneurysms which can bleed causing a potentially fatal subarachnoid haemorrhage. The gene for adult polycystic kidney disease lies on the short arm of chromosome 16 (16p) and has recently been identified, though its function remains unclear. A number of methods are available for genetic diagnosis.

- The identification of a restriction fragment length polymorphism (RFLP) can make the genetic diagnosis of monogenic diseases such as adult polycystic kidney disease relatively straightforward. Restriction enzymes recognize specific DNA sequences and cut the DNA wherever they encounter these sites so producing fragments of DNA of different sizes. Depending on the sequence of the patients DNA, the position of the enzyme cutting sites will vary and so the size of the fragments will vary in a way which distinguishes those carrying the disease gene from those carrying the normal gene.

- The basic method of RFLP diagnosis is as follows. Genomic DNA is cut with a restriction enzyme to produce fragments. As DNA carries a negative charge proportional to its length, the cut fragments can be separated on the basis of their size by electrophoresis in a gel and transferred to a nitrocellulose or nylon membrane by a process known as Southern blotting. The fragment of interest contains the disease gene or a marker which is genetically linked to this gene and so near to it. If part of the sequence of this fragment is known then it can be identified by using a piece of radioactive DNA known as a probe which has a complementary DNA sequence and so binds specifically to the desired fragment on the membrane. In this way the fragment can be identified by the bound radioactivity using autoradiography and its length calculated from the position of the radioactivity on the membrane.

- Single stranded conformational polymorphism (SSCP) is another method for distinguishing genes with different sequences. Double stranded genomic DNA from a patient is cut by restriction enzymes into fragments and denatured to produce single stranded DNA. The mobility of fragments of single stranded DNA in electrophoretic gels is affected by the sequence of the DNA and so disease and normal genes can be distinguished by their different mobilities. The fragment of interest can be identified using a radioactive probe.

- Amplification refractory mutation system–polymerase chain reaction (ARMS–PCR) is another means of genetic diagnosis which relies on the ability of changes in the sequence of the disease gene or a nearby linker to affect the efficiency of a polymerase chain reaction. In this way the amount and size of the DNA amplified by the polymerase chain reaction is determined by the presence or absence of sequences in or near the disease gene. The principle of the polymerase chain reaction is explained in Fig. 6. In the normal gene, two PCR primers of defined sequence may, for example, amplify a 400 base pair (bp) length of DNA. However, in the disease gene, if a mutation occurs in a region normally bound by one of these primers then there will be no polymerase chain reaction and no DNA amplification, thus distinguishing the normal from the disease gene.

• A direct approach to diagnosis is to sequence the patient's genes to see whether they carry the normal or the disease gene. Often this is done after amplification of the relevant gene by a normal polymerase chain reaction.

## 19 F,T,T,T,T

Erythropoeitin promotes red cell production. As the kidney fails, erythropoetin production falls and anaemia results. The kidney excretes phosphate and so phosphate levels accumulate. The accumulation of phosphate can be associated with a tendency to reduced calcium, especially in the context of impaired vitamin D metabolism by the kidney. (The kidney contains a 1-alpha-hydroxylase which converts 25-hydroxy vitamin $D_3$ to 1,25-hydroxy vitamin $D_3$.) The result is a compensatory or secondary hyperparathyroidism which can become tertiary hyperparathyroidism if the parathyroid glands become autonomous. Amyloidosis tend to occur in dialysis patients and is the result of beta-2-microglobulin amyloid deposition. Peptic ulceration is increased and this may be related to high serum gastrin levels as the kidney normally catabolises gastrin.

## 20 T,T,F,T,F

Goodpasture's disease is characterized by the presence of antibodies against the basement membrane in the glomerulus. These antibodies often cross-react with the basement membrane in the lung. The condition can be of rapid onset and is typically characterized by a rapidly progressive glomerulonephritis with necrosis and crescent formation in the glomerulus. In addition, there may be diffuse alveolar haemorrhage which can be fatal. Treatment is with immunosuppression using steroids and cyclophosphamide and often plasma exchange. The condition is more common in men than women and there is a strong association with HLA-DR2. The antigen has been identified as alpha-3-collagen. Curiously, this is absent in Alport's disease which is also a cause of renal failure. If patients with Alport's disease are given a renal transplant, they can develop an immune response to this antigen which they have not previously seen. This can result in antiglomerular basement membrane antibody disease in the transplanted kidney.

# Neurology

## 1 T,T,F,F,T

The spinal cord ends above L2, so lumbar puncture is performed below this level. The blood supply to the brain is illustrated in Fig. 9. The brain derives its blood supply from the internal carotid and vertebral arteries. The internal carotid artery divides into the anterior and middle cerebral arteries which together supply the anterior–superior two thirds of the brain.

- The anterior cerebral artery supplies much of the frontal and parietal cortices.
- The middle cerebral artery supplies the basal ganglia, internal capsule, and large areas of the frontal, parietal, temporal and anterior occipital cortex.
- The two vertebral arteries arise from the subclavian arteries and join to form a basilar artery which divides into two posterior cerebral arteries to supply the posterior inferior brain.

In both the sympathetic and parasympathetic system fibres leaving the central nervous system first synapse in a ganglion, then postganglionic fibres pass to the innervated organ.

Neurology • **Answers**

- In the parasympathetic system, the neurotransmitter is acetylcholine in both the terminal ganglion and in the final synapse with the innervated organ.
- In the sympathetic system the ganglion is usually para or prevertebral; as in the parasympathetic system the ganglionic

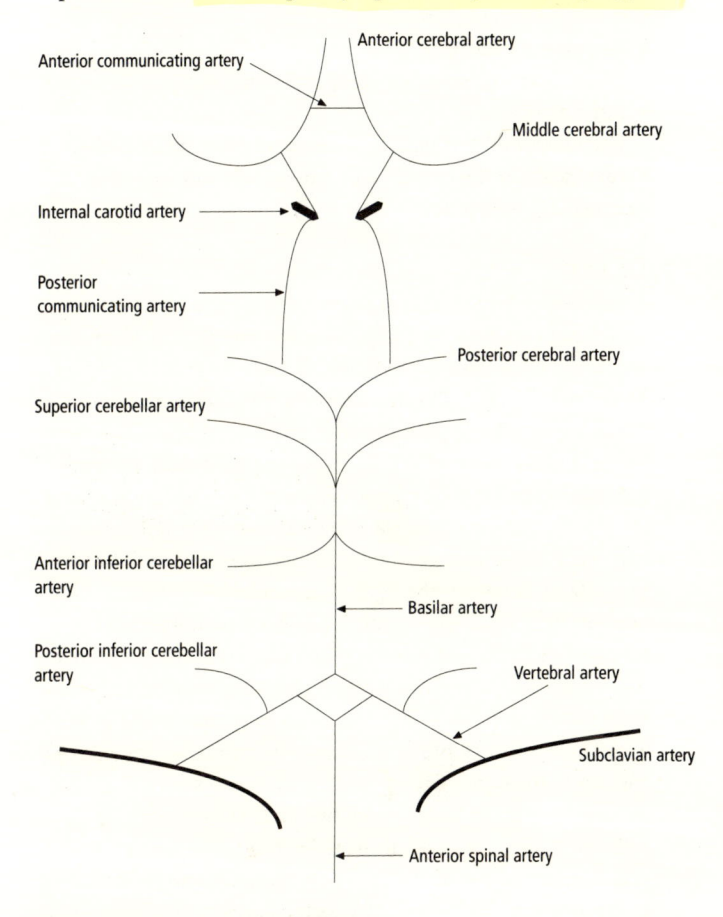

**Figure 9** The blood supply of the brain.

**Answers** • Neurology

neurotransmitter is acetylcholine but the final synapse is noradrenergic.

## 2 T,T,T,T,T

The effects of vitamin $B_{12}$ deficiency are varied, but in the nervous system important features are:
- peripheral neuropathy
- myelopathy (disease of the spinal cord) and
- optic atrophy.

The neuropathy is usually a distal sensory neuropathy. Paraesthesia in the presence of a megaloblastic anaemia suggests $B_{12}$ deficiency.

## 3 T,T,T,F,F

A number of large well conducted trials have produced important conclusions concerning the prevention of strokes and these have been well reviewed (*New England Journal of Medicine* 1995; **332**: 238–48). Both aspirin and warfarin reduce the risk of stroke in patients with atrial fibrillation, warfarin being slightly more effective. However, for young patients the risk of stroke under these circumstances is very low and for elderly patients the risk of an adverse drug reaction is high so in these two groups there may be no overall benefit. In contrast, between the ages of around 60–75, there is clear benefit. In several trials benefit has been demonstrated in terms of reduction of strokes when carotid endarterectomy was compared to medical therapy, but this was only the case with severe stenosis (>70% stenosis) in symptomatic patients. Two large primary prevention studies examined the use of aspirin in male physicians. In the American study at a dose of 325 mg/day there was a reduction in first myocardial infarction, but not in death from stroke. In the British study, which used a dose of 500 mg/day, there was no reduction in death from stroke. Systolic hypertension is a more powerful risk factor than diastolic hypertension.

## 4 T,T,T,T,T

Prions are small proteinacious infectious particles not destroyed by procedures damaging nucleic acids and so not containing DNA. They contain a prion protein known as PrPsc which is an abnormal isoform of the cellular protein PrPc generated by a post translational process (after protein synthesis) from a gene on human chromosome 20. It seems likely that the abnormal form of the protein is infectious and can cause a conformational change in the normal protein, making it like itself and so propagating itself. Creutzfeldt–Jakob disease can be transmitted by human material such as pituitary extracts used to treat growth hormone deficiency, but most cases are sporadic with around 10% of cases inherited in an autosomal dominant manner. On histological examination of the brain, most prion diseases show vacuolation and proliferation of fibrous astrocytes or astrocytic gliosis. Amyloid deposition is common. The clinical course in Creutzfeldt–Jakob disease invariably ends in death after a period of rapid, severe neurological decline with dementia. Kuru is a fatal form of cerebellar ataxia presumed to result from a transmissible prion occurring in and confined to the Fore tribe in New Guinea. Transmission is believed to occur as a result of ingestion of the brain of an affected individual.

## 5 T,T,F,T,T

The key risk factors are hypertension, previous transient ischaemic attack, atrial fibrillation, peripheral vascular disease, carotid stenosis, and a high haematocrit. Other factors include alcohol, lipids, smoking and, in middle aged women, the contraceptive pill. Left atrial myxoma can cause embolic stroke. Antiphospholipid syndrome increases the risk of cerebral thrombosis.

**Answers** • Neurology

**6 F,T,T,F,T**

The characteristic pathological change in multiple sclerosis is the white matter plaque which is an area of central demyelination. Peripheral demyelination is not a feature of multiple sclerosis. Vulnerable sites include the optic nerve, brainstem, spinal cord and periventricular regions, but all areas can be affected. The concordance rate in monozygotic twins is 25–30% compared with 2–5% in dizygotic twins. There are HLA associations with class II haplotypes DRw15 and DQw6, but a number of genome wide searches have suggested that other genetic loci play a role. The appearances on magnetic resonance imaging is not specific, but in the appropriate clinical setting can confirm a diagnosis of multiple sclerosis and is a sensitive index of disease activity. Optic neuritis is common and the residual effects of demyelination are a slowing of the visual evoked potential.

**7 T,F,T,F,F**

The main causes of peripheral nerve thickening are leprosy, amyloidosis, trauma and some forms of hereditary motor and sensory neuropathies.

**8 T,F,T,T,T**

The dorsal columns are on the posterior aspect of the spinal cord and carry large myelinated nerve fibres. Fibres pass from the dorsal root ganglion to the ipsilateral dorsal column and pass up the spine and cross in the medulla. They are therefore ipsilateral in the cord, the left column carrying fibres from the left side of the body. They principally transmit joint position sense and light touch sensation. The spinothalamic tract carries pain and temperature sensation. The main diseases which affect the dorsal columns are:
- tabes dorsalis (syphilis)
- vitamin $B_{12}$ deficiency (subacute combined degeneration of the cord)

Neurology • **Answers**

- Friedreich's ataxia (an inherited spinocerebellar degeneration)
- multiple sclerosis
- diabetes – rarely.

## 9 T,T,T,T,T

A mononeuritis multiplex is a neuropathy affecting several different nerves simultaneously. The main causes are polyarteritis nodosa, leprosy, diabetes, sarcoidosis and amyloidosis. Other causes include neurofibromatosis and malignancy associated neuropathy. In polyarteritis nodosa there may be a vasculitis affecting the vessels supplying the peripheral nerves.

## 10 T,F,F,T,T

The combination of upgoing plantars and absent tendon reflexes can occur where there is both lower and upper motor neurone damage; upper motor neurone damage causes the upgoing plantar and lower motor neurone damage causes the absent reflex. Combined damage to the upper and lower motor neurones can occur in motor neurone disease. In vitamin $B_{12}$ deficiency damage to the corticospinal tracts can occur in the presence of a peripheral neuropathy. Friedreich's ataxia is an autosomal recessive disorder associated with spinocerebellar degeneration and reduced tendon reflexes. Other causes can include spinal shock and a conus medullaris lesion.

## 11 F,T,F,F,F

Diphtheria toxin affects protein synthesis and can result in segmental demyelination. A distal motor neuropathy can result, but more commonly palatal weakness occurs. Leprosy causes sensory loss. In hereditary motor and sensory neuropathy or Charcot–Marie–Tooth disease, acute intermittent porphyria and Guillain–Barré syndrome there may be sen-

## Answers • Neurology

sory loss but motor changes predominate. The main causes of a predominantly sensory neuropathy are:
- diabetes;
- leprosy;
- amyloidosis;
- malignancy related neuropathy and
- vitamin $B_{12}$ deficiency.

The main causes of a predominantly motor neuropathy are:
- hereditary motor and sensory neuropathy or Charcot–Marie–Tooth disease;
- acute intermittent porphyria;
- Guillain–Barré syndrome;
- diphtheria and
- lead toxicity.

In amyloidosis, sensory neuropathy can precede motor neuropathy.

## 12 T,T,F,T,T

Myasthaenia gravis is an autoimmune disease in which there is impaired function of the acetylcholine receptor. In many cases antibodies to this receptor are present and are thought to be involved in the pathogenesis of the disease. Thymic hyperplasia is common and thymomas occur in about 10% of cases. Thymectomy may improve those patients without thymoma. In contrast, in the presence of a thymoma it is necessary to perform thymectomy to treat the tumour but this does not usually help the myaesthaenia. Inhibition of acetylcholinesterase by edrophonium bromide is a diagnostic test, resulting in a temporary improvement in cholinergic transmission. Inhibition of acetylcholinesterase by pyridostigmine is used as a treatment and improves symptoms but does not alter the natural history of the disease. Immunosuppression may be of benefit in the long term. Clinical features include ptosis, diplopia and fatiguability on testing muscle power.

### 13 T,F,F,F,F

Lewy bodies are eosinophilic cytoplasmic inclusions and are characteristic of the histological appearance of Parkinson's disease which affects the substantia nigra of the basal ganglia. The disease causes degeneration of dopaminergic neurones, especially those projecting from the substantia nigra to the striatum (the caudate nucleus and the putamen). Consequently there is dopamine deficiency in the affected pathways. The key clinical features are the triad of tremor, rigidity and akinesia. The tremor is worse at rest. Bladder and bowel dysfunction resulting in constipation and urinary retention are common and often resistant to treatment. Intellectual function may deteriorate and dementia can occur.

### 14 T,T,T,F,T

Sumatriptan is a 5-hydroxytryptamine (5-HT) agonist which causes vasoconstriction at 5-HT1 receptors and this is probably the mechanism of action in migraine. It is thought that with migraine there is initial vasoconstriction, sometimes associated with ischaemic features and then this is followed by vasodilatation which causes the headache. Sumatriptan by causing vasoconstriction may attenuate the vasodilatory headache phase. Tricyclic antidepressants inhibit the reuptake of both 5-HT and noradrenaline, but the selective 5-HT reuptake inhibitors such as fluoxetine, fluvoxamine, paroxetine and sertraline only inhibit the reuptake of 5-HT. Ondansetron, an antiemetic is an antagonist at 5-HT3 receptors and blocks a vomiting reflex.

### 15 T,T,T,T,T

Vitamin $B_1$ (Thiamine) deficiency occurs in malnutrition or chronic alcoholics. Glucose metabolism is impaired with the

accumulation of pyruvate and lactate. Heart failure can result in severe cases. The principal neurological changes include a symmetrical polyneuropathy or Wernicke–Korsakoff's syndrome which is reversible if treated early, but can become irreversible if left untreated. Wernicke–Korsakoff's syndrome consists of a triad of
- eye signs,
- ataxia and
- confusion.

The commonest eye signs are nystagmus, ocular palsies or defects of conjugate gaze; the confusion typically includes amnesia especially for recent events. Treatment is with thiamine. If glucose is given without thiamine, the patients cannot deal with the glucose load and rapid deterioration and death can occur.

### 16 T,T,T,T,F

*Borrelia burgdorferei* is a spirochaete transmitted by ixodid ticks and the disease is known as Lyme disease. The first stage consists of the characteristic rash, erythema chronicum migrans, malaise, lymphadenopathy and arthralgia. In the second stage cranial or peripheral neuropathies and myocarditis can occur. A chronic relapsing arthritis has been reported as the third stage. The diagnosis is usually made serologically and treatment is with penicillin.

### 17 T,F,T,F,F

Charcot–Marie–Tooth disease is a form of hereditary sensory and motor neuropathy characterized by distal weakness and often atrophy hence the synonym peroneal muscular atrophy. Duchenne muscular dystrophy is an X-linked disorder characterized by proximal muscle weakness and wasting. Dystrophia myotonica is an autosomal dominant condition carried on chromosome 19. Features include a distal weakness, myotonia, frontal baldness, cataracts, low intelligence, cardiomyopathy and glucose intolerance. Wilson's disease is an autosomal recessive inborn error of copper metabolism resulting in copper deposition in certain tissues. This results in liver disease, Kayser–Fleischer rings in the eyes and degeneration of the basal ganglia causing akinesia, rigidity and eventually dementia. Huntington's disease is an autosomal dominant condition characterized by chorea often with personality changes which progresses to dementia. This disease is associated with the trinucleotide repeat (CAG) on chromosome 4; an increased number of repeats occurs in the disease compared to normal patients.

## 18 F,F,T,T,T

In the pupillary light reflex, afferent impulses travel along the optic nerve to the lateral geniculate bodies and then to the Edinger–Westphal nucleus. Efferent fibres travel from this nucleus in the third nerve to the ciliary ganglion from which postganglionic fibres pass to the sphincter pupillae which controls pupil dilatation. This is shown schematically in Fig. 10. Neurones in the brainstem are involved in this reflex, but the occipital cortex is not involved and so not necessary for an intact pupillary reflex. In the doll's eye (oculo–cephalic) reflex, the head is rapidly rotated sideways then held still. If the brainstem is intact, afferent impulses from the vestibular apparatus pass in the eighth nerve to the vestibular nuclei. Fibres from the vestibular nuclei travel via the medial longitudinal fasciculus to the nuclei of the third, fourth and sixth nerves, from where efferent fibres pass to the rectus muscles controlling eye movement. In an unconscious patient, the eyes initially do not move with the head, but lag behind then catch up – this is the doll's head reflex. Damage to the brainstem can destroy this reflex so that the eyes stay fixed with respect to the head. The afferent of the corneal reflex is the fifth nerve (trigeminal) and the efferent the seventh nerve (facial). Cocaine dilates normal pupils, whereas opiates constrict them.

## 19  T,T,T,T,F

Normal cerebrospinal fluid contains 0.15–0.5 g/l of total protein and usually no more than five lymphocytes or mononuclear cells per microlitre (= mm$^3$). Any central nervous system disease or meningeal disease can increase the cell count or protein count.

• With bacterial infection the predominant cells are usually neutrophils.

• The main causes of a predominantly lymphocytic picture are viral infection, syphilis, tuberculosis, cryptococcus, sarcoidosis and leukaemia.

In motor neurone disease, the cerebrospinal fluid protein is raised in about 20% of cases, but there is no increase in cell count.

## 20  T,F,T,T,T

The visual pathway is shown in Fig. 10. The lateral retina in the left eye and the medial retina in the right eye view the right visual field. Fibres from these two regions join after the fibres from the medial right retina have crossed the midline in the optic chiasm. Fibres supplying the upper visual field pass to the occipital cortex via the temporal lobe and those from the lower visual field pass to the occipital cortex via the parietal lobe.

• Therefore, lesions in the temporal cortex cause loss of the upper quadrant of the visual field and lesions in the parietal cortex cause loss of the lower quadrant of the visual field.

• Lesions of the dominant temporal lobe can damage Wernicke's area causing a receptive dysphasia, lesions of the frontal lobe can damage Broca's area producing an expressive dysphasia.

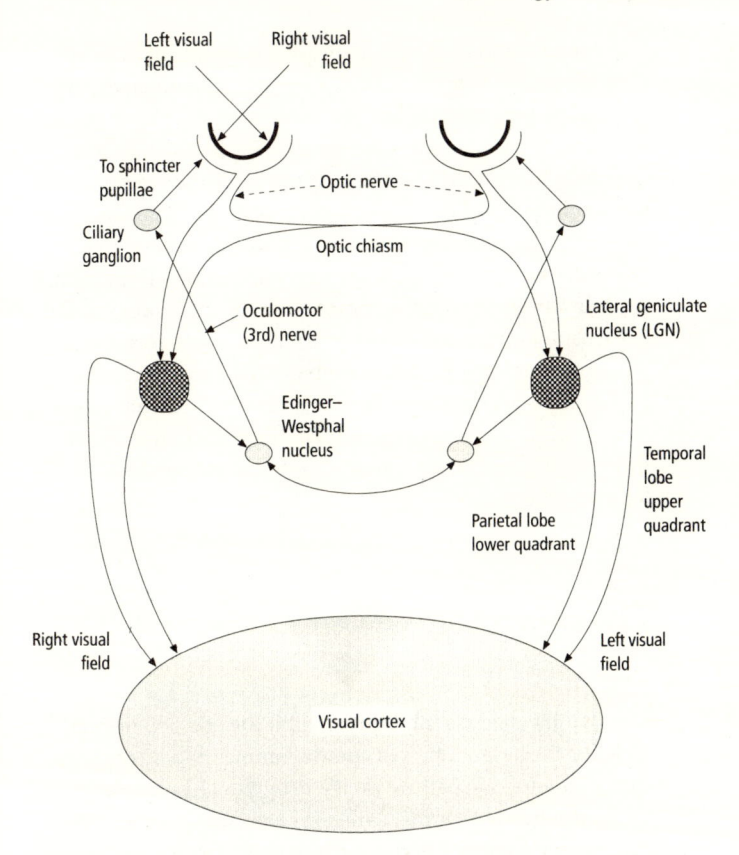

**Figure 10** The visual pathways. A schematic view of the visual pathway from above. Considering the left visual field, images from this field are received by the right sides of both retina and pass in the optic nerve, where impulses from the left eye cross the optic chiasm and fibres from both eyes pass to the lateral geniculate nucleus. From there fibres from the upper field pass through the temporal lobe and fibres from the lower field pass through the parietal lobe to reach the visual cortex. The light reflex does not pass through the visual cortex.

### Answers • Neurology/Pharmacology

In broad terms, a receptive dysphasia results in difficulty with the comprehension of language, whereas in an expressive dysphasia, the problem lies more with the motor control of language production. With an anterior cerebral artery occlusion there is a severe loss of function in the leg because the leg motor (and usually sensory) cortex is damaged. However, the arm and face may be affected, usually to a lesser degree by damage to the internal capsule. The internal capsule carries descending fibres from the motor cortex. The corticospinal tract carries fibres from the motor cortex and passes through the posterior limb of the internal capsule, eventually forming the pyramids in the medulla and crossing at this point. Damage to the tract in the midbrain is above this crossing and so can cause a contralateral paralysis of the leg and arm.

# Pharmacology

### 1 T,F,F,T,F

Monoamine oxidase inhibitors inhibit the enzyme responsible for the degradation of catecholamines and so enhance catecholaminergic pathways. If a drug which enhances these pathways by another mechanism is also administered, life threatening hypertension can result from excess catecholaminergic activity. Such drugs include pethidine, tricyclic antidepressants, sympathomimetic amines, such as pseudoephedrine in cough remedies. If a supply of amine rich food, such as cheese, which contains tyramine is given, a similar outcome can occur. The tyramine is not degraded by peripheral monoamine oxidases because of the drug inhibition and causes the release of catecholamines from sympathetic neurones and the adrenal medulla. Selegiline preferentially inhibits monoamine oxidase B and is of use in Parkinson's disease.

### 2 T,T,F,F,T

5-hydroxytryptamine (5-HT) is the same as serotonin. There are a number of different receptor types, not all of which have clearly recognized functions or clinical relevance.

- 5-HT1 agonists, such as sumatriptan, are of benefit in migraine where they inhibit the dilatation of intracranial vessels which is associated with the headache. This dilatation usually follows a period of vasoconstriction. Sumatriptan can produce a degree of coronary vasoconstriction which can be a problem in the presence of pre-existing coronary artery disease.
- The 5-HT reuptake inhibitors such as paroxetine, fluoxetine and fluvoxamine block the reuptake of 5-HT at neuronal synapses.
- Ondansetron is an antagonist at 5-HT3 receptors and is of use as an antiemetic with chemotherapy.

### 3 T,T,F,T,T

Cocaine enhances certain catecholaminergic pathways and may directly act on smooth muscle to cause vasoconstriction. Enhanced catecholaminergic transmission is associated with pupillary dilatation which can occur when cocaine has been used. The sympathetic system dilates the pupils and the parasympathetic system constricts them. There are now numerous reports of cocaine related myocardial infarction in the absence of significant coronary artery disease. Overdose can cause medullary stimulation with hypertension, tachycardia and subsequently convulsions and dysrhythmias. Chronic nasal administration can produce septal perforation, possibly brought about by repeated vasospasm and ischaemic damage to the tissues. Crack is cocaine which has

### Answers • Pharmacology

been separated from its hydrochloride salt and so can be vaporized and inhaled into the lungs for rapid absorption.

### 4 T,T,F,T,F

Adenosine is an endogenous nucleoside that stimulates an outward potassium current in supraventricular tissue, causing the hyperpolarization of atrial cells. Atrioventricular nodal block can occur transiently and these effects contribute to its action in terminating supraventricular tachydysrhythmias. Aminophylline antagonizes the effects of adenosine. In asthmatics, bronchospasm can be precipitated by adenosine. A broad complex tachycardia can result from a supraventricular or ventricular tachycardia. Adenosine does not usually cardiovert ventricular dysrhythmias, but its action is very short lived and it does not do any harm. In contrast, a calcium channel blocker will not usually stop a ventricular dysrhythmia, but its effect is longer lasting and can cause haemodynamic collapse, especially if there is a markedly negative inotropic action.

### 5 T,F,F,F,F

Nitric oxide is a vasodilator produced from L-arginine by a constitutive enzyme in the vascular endothelium and by an inducible enzyme expressed throughout the vessel wall in response to endotoxin and cytokines. Activity of the constitutive enzyme may play a role in the normal control of vessel tone and so of blood pressure. Expression of the inducible enzyme leads to the production of large quantities of nitric oxide and vasodilatation. In severe infection, this may contribute to haemodynamic collapse which is often seen. The half life is very short, of the order of a few seconds. There are inhibitors of nitric oxide synthesis such as L-N-monomethyl-L-arginine (L-NMMA) which have been studied in conditions such as septic shock.

Pharmacology • **Answers**

## 6 T,T,T,F,F

Sulphonylureas stimulate insulin secretion and may enhance the peripheral response to insulin. Lactic acidosis is a particular problem when metformin is given in the presence of renal impairment. The Diabetes Control and Complications Trial (DCCT) demonstrated that tight control did reduce the frequency of microvascular complications in insulin dependent diabetes mellitus, but increased the incidence of hypoglycaemia (*New England Journal of Medicine* 1994; 329: 977–86). The avoidance of obesity and regular exercise make control easier. Dietary control is essential whatever drug therapy is used and may reduce drug requirements.

## 7 T,F,T,F,F

Platelet aggregation is promoted by thromboxanes which are produced by platelets and is inhibited by prostacyclins which are produced by the endothelium. Aspirin acts by inhibiting cyclo-oxygenase, an enzyme involved in the synthesis of both of these factors, but the endothelium, unlike platelets has a nucleus and so can produce new cyclo-oxygenase. The overall effect is a net inhibition of thromboxane production by the endothelium, and so an inhibition of platelet aggregation. von Willebrand factor is required for the adherence of platelets to exposed subendothelial tissue following damage to the endothelium.

## 8 F,F,F,T,F

Uric acid undergoes net renal excretion by a process of filtration, tubular secretion and tubular reabsorption. Gout may occur when there is an accumulation of uric acid either because of a reduced capacity for urinary excretion or because of increased production, such as that associated with the cellular destruction of cancer chemotherapy. The accumulated urate can crystallize and trigger inflammation.

### Answers • Pharmacology

Colchicine, unlike nonsteroidal anti-inflammatory drugs can reasonably be used in patients with renal failure. Allopurinol inhibits the synthesis of uric acid from xanthine and of xanthine from hypoxanthine. Allopurinol inhibits the enzymatic oxidation of azathioprine and its metabolite mercaptopurine and this can cause excessive immunosuppression from the high effective dose of azathioprine which results. Nonsteroidal anti-inflammatory drugs are routinely used for the treatment of acute gout and can be used in patients on allopurinol. Thiazide diuretics can increase urate levels and precipitate gout and for this reason are best avoided.

### 9 T,T,T,T,T

Most drugs used to combat cancer act either by a hormonal mechanism or a cytotoxic action. Cytotoxic drugs usually act by one or more of the following mechanisms: interference with the production of DNA, disruption to already formed DNA or damage to the mitotic spindle apparatus. These effects have some selectivity for rapidly dividing cells and so tend to affect the gut, bone marrow and hair follicles. For this reason, almost all cytotoxic drugs can cause bone marrow suppression, hair loss, nausea and vomiting and general immunosuppression, but certain specific side-effects are well recognized. The chances of haemorrhagic cystitis occurring with cyclophosphamide can be minimized by coadministration of mesna and maintenance of good hydration and urine output. Mesna reacts in the urine with the cyclophosphamide metabolite acrolein which is responsible for the haemorrhagic cystitis. The dilated cardiomyopathy associated with adriamycin can be a late occurrence and is probably related to total dose. Cisplatin nephrotoxicity is reduced by adequate hydration and possibly by the coadministration of cimetidine and verapamil.

Pharmacology • **Answers**

## 10 T,T,T,F,T

Co-trimoxazole is trimethoprim and sulphamethoxazole and is of prophylactic value for *Pneumocystis carinii* in advanced HIV infection and in immunosuppressed patients such as those with transplants. Aspirin is of value in the prevention of secondary and probably primary myocardial infarction. Ondansetron is a specific 5-HT3 antagonist and is useful in the prevention of drug induced vomiting. Pyridoxine, not isoniazid is used to reduce the incidence of isoniazid induced peripheral neuropathy. Travellers diarrhoea is commonly caused by *Escherichia coli* strains and is reduced by administration of various antibiotics, such as cotrimoxazole or ciprofloxacin.

## 11 F,T,T,F,T

Thiazide diuretics can cause impaired glucose tolerance and may worsen glycaemic control in diabetics. It is said that beta blockers may reduce the awareness of hypoglycaemic symptoms. Reasonable choices in diabetes would be angiotensin converting enzyme inhibitors or calcium channel antagonists. In a patient with chronic renal failure on dialysis, angiotensin converting enzyme inhibitors can safely be used and may be of benefit if renin secretion from non-functional kidneys is a contributory factor in the hypertension. Labetalol is generally safe in pregnancy as is nifedipine. Both have also been used during breastfeeding. Beta blockers such as nifedipine can worsen the symptoms of peripheral vascular insufficiency.

## 12 F,T,F,T,F

Rifampicin induces hepatic enzymes and can increase the metabolism of oral contraceptive drugs, so reducing their efficacy. Frusemide is a potassium wasting diuretic, whereas triamterene is a potassium conserving diuretic and for this reason the two are often combined in a single preparation.

**Answers** • Pharmacology

Generally speaking, there is reduced dopaminergic transmission in Parkinson's disease and enhanced dopaminergic activity in schizophrenia. Chlorpromazine has an antidopaminergic effect, whereas L-dopa enhances dopaminergic transmission in Parkinson's disease. Chlorpromazine can worsen extra-pyramidal motor symptoms in Parkinson's disease and L-dopa is usually avoided in schizophrenia. Bronchodilation is mediated by beta-2 agonists. Adrenaline and dopamine are both positive inotropes and low dose dopamine is often coadministered with adrenaline to maintain renal and gut blood flow by vasodilation in these regions. Although salbutamol is a beta-2 agonist and atenolol a beta-1 antagonist, nevertheless, the selectivity of atenolol is not complete and like most other beta blockers atenolol can antagonize beta-2 receptors, thus reducing the effect of salbutamol and resulting in worse bronchoconstriction.

### 13 T,F,F,T,F

Acyclovir specifically inhibits the viral, but not the human thymidine kinase enzyme, hence its selective toxicity to the virus. Ampicillin and penicillin based antibiotics inhibit bacterial cell wall synthesis, not protein synthesis. Pyridostigmine acts by inhibiting acetylcholine esterase, the enzyme which degrades acetylcholine and this action enhances cholinergic transmission. Atropine inhibits cholinergic transmission at muscarinic receptors and so blocks parasympathetic transmission. This can result in reduced secretions, pupillary dilatation and an accelerated heart rate.

### 14 T,T,T,T,F

Total parenteral nutrition is used in patients who cannot be fed enterally and necessitates venous cannulation, usually of the subclavian or internal jugular veins. The risks of central venous cannulation include bleeding, arterial puncture and pneumothorax. In addition, there is a risk of air embolus

Pharmacology • **Answers**

during insertion of the catheter and when the associated bags or tubing are replaced. Infection is always a possibility when there is an indwelling venous cannula. Elevations of bilirubin, alkaline phosphatase, lactate dehydrogenase and hepatic transaminases are common in patients on total parenteral nutrition. When liver biopsies have been performed on patients with abnormal liver function on total parenteral nutrition, peripheral fatty changes have been observed, but the exact aetiology of these changes is unclear. Hypoglycaemia can occur for various reasons, especially if insulin production or sensitivity is impaired and parenteral glucose input is high. If phosphate intake in the feed is too low then hypophosphataemia can occur. In type I hyperlipidaemia chylomicrons are elevated and as they result from the digestion of lipids in the gut, their elevation is certainly not a feature of total parenteral nutrition.

The World Health Organization classification of hyperlipidaemias is based on the plasma lipoprotein abnormalities and is given below as are the effects on plasma cholesterol and triglycerides. Chylomicrons and very low density lipoprotein (VLDL) principally contain triglycerides, low density lipoprotein (LDL) and high density lipoprotein (HDL) principally contain cholesterol and intermediate density lipoproteins (IDL) contain both cholesterol and triglycerides.

- Type I results from lipoprotein lipase deficiency and is associated with excess chylomicrons and causes raised plasma triglycerides.
- Type IIa (familial hypercholesterolaemia) is dominant and results from LDL receptor mutations causing excess LDL. Tendon xanthomas can occur and plasma cholesterol is raised.
- Type IIb (combined familial hyperlipidaemia) is usually a dominant condition and raises both plasma cholesterol and triglycerides. Usually both LDL and VLDL are elevated.

### Answers • Pharmacology

- Type III (remnant hyperlipoproteinaemia) is recessive and is associated with the homozygosity for the apoE2 allele leading to excess IDL. Both plasma cholesterol and triglycerides are raised and there is an association with palmar xanthoma.
- Type IV (familial hypertriglyeridaemia) is usually a dominant disorder associated with raised VLDL, impaired glucose tolerance, obesity, eruptive xanthomas, pancreatitis and markedly raised plasma triglycerides.
- Type V has features in common with both types I and IV and causes hypertriglyceridaemia.

### 15 T,F,T,T,F

Bronchodilation is mediated by beta-2 adrenoreceptors and salbutamol is a beta-2 selective agonist. Mefenamic acid inhibits prostaglandin synthesis and is used for relief of dysmenorrhoea. At low doses dopamine acts principally on dopaminergic receptors, but at higher doses has effects on both beta-1 and alpha receptors. Dopamine acts on D1 (dopaminergic) and on D2 receptors. D1 receptors mediate smooth muscle relaxation in the gut and kidney; D2 receptors occupy a presynaptic site and oppose noradrenaline release. Beta-1 adrenergic agonists such as dobutamine have a positive inotropic and chronotropic action. Atenolol is a beta-1 blocker and so can impair bronchodilation and worsen asthma. Isoprenaline is a beta-agonist and typically causes tachycardia.

### 16 T,T,T,T,F

Paracetamol is an inhibitor of prostaglandin synthesis. A proportion of the drug is metabolized by cytochrome P-450 dependent oxidases to a toxic metabolite. This metabolite is detoxified by conjugation with glutathione and excreted by the kidney. In overdose, glutathione becomes depleted and the toxic metabolite accumulates and binds sulphydryl

Pharmacology • **Answers**

groups in hepatic intracellular proteins causing hepatocyte death. *N*-acetyl-cysteine is metabolized to cysteine, a glutathione precursor to replenish glutathione supplies. Impaired clotting – usually seen first as a rise in prothrombin time is an early marker of liver damage in paracetamol overdose.

### 17 T,T,T,T,T

Bumetanide, like the other loop diuretics is a well recognized cause of renal potassium wasting. Most corticosteroids such as triamcinolone and prednisolone have some mineralocorticoid activity stimulating sodium retention and potassium excretion, which occurs principally in the distal tubule. Adenyl cyclase promotes the production of cAMP and phosphodiesterase promotes the degradation of cAMP. Within tubular cells, cAMP promotes potassium transport into the tubules and so increases renal potassium excretion.

- Aminophylline is a phosphodiesterase inhibitor and causes an elevation in intracellular cAMP and so potassium loss.
- Salbutamol, like other beta-agonists activates adenyl cyclase resulting in intracellular accumulation of cAMP and so potassium wasting.

### 18 T,T,T,T,T

The response of any patient to any drug can always be idiosyncratic and as a general principle any drug could cause any adverse reaction. Nevertheless, certain drugs have a propensity to cause specific adverse reactions. Erythema multiforme is a rash of target-like lesions and in extreme cases is associated with involvement of the mouth, genitalia and sometimes even the eyes. Amiodarone can result in a dark discolouration of sun exposed skin. The commonest skin reaction to drugs is a toxic erythema with macular or maculopapular lesions, sometimes with an urticarial element.

## Answers • Pharmacology

Erythema nodosum is well recognized in the presence of synthetic oestrogens or sulphonamides, but can also occur in the presence of sarcoidosis, inflammatory bowel disease or mycobacterial infection. Gold therapy can cause proteinuria, membranous nephropathy, blood disorders, rashes and diarrhoea.

### 19 T,T,T,F,T

Frusemide, like the other loop diuretics, causes enhanced renal excretion of sodium and chloride. This is particularly so in oedema states such as heart failure, where natriuretic regulation is already impaired and hyponatraemia frequently results. Carbamazepine and chlorpropamide can both result in a syndrome of inappropriate antidiuretic hormone secretion (SIADH). The excess antidiuretic hormone causes hyponatraemia by excessive water retention which is not balanced by salt retention. Mineralocorticoids, such as fludrocortisone promote sodium retention and potassium excretion in the distal tubule. Aminoglutethimide is sometimes used when there is excess cortisol production. It inhibits the first step in steroid synthesis which is the conversion of cholesterol to pregnenolone and so inhibits the production of all endogenous steroids. The result of this is a reduction in all steroid activity, including mineralocorticoid activity and consequently hyponatraemia can occur. It is usual for this reason to coadminister supplementary corticosteroid and mineralocorticoid to prevent an Addisonian crisis of steroid deficiency with hypovolaemia, hyponatraemia and hypoglycaemia.

### 20 F,T,T,F,T

Aspirin overdose can initially cause a respiratory alkalosis by stimulating respiratory effort and so lowering plasma carbon dioxide levels. This is usually followed by a metabolic acidosis as the drug itself is acidic and uncouples mitochondrial oxidative phosphorylation and influences other metabolic pathways allowing lactic acid and ketones to accumulate. Phenytoin has a class I antiarrhythmic action, but like any antiarrhythmic, can itself cause dysrhythmias, especially in overdose. Digoxin slows atrioventricular nodal conduction causing heart block, but overdose can cause other dysrhythmias. Amitriptylline overdose typically results in fitting and dysrhythmias. Azathioprine can certainly cause neutropaenia, even at normal doses in susceptible individuals.

# Respiratory

### 1 T,T,F,T,T

Gas transfer is measured by the removal of carbon monoxide (CO) from the inhaled gas. When corrected for ventilated volume, the result is known as the gas transfer coefficient (KCO). In Goodpasture's syndrome alveolar haemorrhage occurs and haemoglobin in this blood avidly absorbs carbon monoxide giving a falsely high gas transfer coefficient. In asthma, airways inflammation can increase blood flow and so removal of CO with a slight rise in KCO. During inspiration, intrathoracic pressure is low and as the chest expands so intrathoracic airways are stretched open and intrathoracic obstruction diminishes. With extrathoracic obstruction, a strong negative pressure must be developed during inspiration which tends to close down the airway, so worsening any obstruction; during expiration the high pressure generated because of the obstruction tends to open the airways so reducing the obstruction. As a flow volume loop distinguishes inspiratory and expiratory air flow, these two types of obstruction can also be distinguished. With emphysema, small airways lose the elastic support of the surrounding lung which normally holds them open and so they close earlier in expiration causing gas trapping and increased residual volume.

## 2 T,F,T,T,F

The central problem in asthma is small airways inflammation which causes airway narrowing with excessive secretion and some bronchospasm. Bronchial hyper responsiveness to exogenous stimuli is usual. An allergic cause in adult asthma occur only in a minority of patients. Churg–Strauss syndrome consists of asthma, eosinophilia and systemic vasculitis. Drugs such as salbutamol, aminophylline and steroids all tend to lower potassium.

## 3 T,F,F,F,F

If previous BCG vaccination has not been given, a positive Heaf test is consistent with active tuberculosis, though not diagnostic as it could represent previous exposure. Occasionally, in overwhelming tuberculosis infection, or in the presence of immunosuppression, the Heaf test may become negative. The Heaf test and Mantoux test are equivalent, but the Heaf test is highly standardized and employs multiple skin pricks. Apical calcification is typical of old tuberculosis and does not imply activity. A three month course of ethambutol alone is inadequate treatment for tuberculosis, but a cough alone is not a diagnostic feature of tuberculosis anyway. Granulomas in tuberculosis are typically caseating and acid-fast bacilli stain with the Ziehl–Nielsen stain. Congo red stains amyloid, which is a rare and late complication of tuberculosis, but does not imply anything about current activity.

## 4 T,F,T,T,T

Urinary calcium excretion may be elevated as may serum calcium as a result of excessive vitamin D production by macrophages in the granulomas. Gallium scanning may highlight areas of activity, which often include lacrimal and parotid glands. Sarcoidosis like any other interstitial lung disease damages the lungs and reduces their ability to exchange gas, so reducing KCO. Imaging of the lung by conventional radiography or computed tomography often shows characteristic changes such as bilateral hilar lymphadenopathy in the early stages or mid-zone fibrosis in advanced cases.

## 5 T,T,T,T,T

Fallot's tetralogy consists of:
- pulmonary stenosis;
- a ventricular septal defect;
- an overriding aorta and
- right ventricular hypertrophy.

A left to right shunt can develop causing hypoxia. Polio may paralyse the muscles of respiration and in the long term may lead to thoracic deformity and a restrictive defect. In ankylosing spondylitis the spinal curvature can produce a restrictive lung defect and in addition upper zone lung fibrosis can occur. Exposure to inorganic dust such as silica in the ceramic industry may cause pulmonary fibrosis with a classic eggshell pattern of calcification on the chest radiograph.

## 6 F,T,T,F,F

Lung disease in coal miners is produced by the inhalation of coal dust and is exacerbated by cigarette smoking. Melanoptysis can occur and is the expectoration of coal material. Caplan's syndrome may occur in miners with rheumatoid arthritis and is the development of round fibrotic nodules in a peripheral distribution. Progressive massive fibrosis can occur when large areas of fibrosis develop, usually in the upper lobes. Cavitation of these areas can cause melanoptysis.

## Answers • Respiratory

### 7 T,T,F,T,T

A pleural effusion with a protein concentration of <30g/l is generally termed a transudate and one with a protein concentration of >30 g/l an exudate. Typically, inflammatory disorders cause exudates whereas transudates occur in conditions associated with peripheral oedema, with or without hypoalbuminaemia. In rheumatoid arthritis, malignancy or infection the high cellular activity results in a low glucose concentration in the effusion. Constrictive pericarditis can cause transudates as can hypoalbuminaemia.

### 8 T,T,F,F,T

Because of the nonlinear shape of the haemoglobin dissociation curve with oxygen, increased ventilation does not increase arterial oxygenation proportionately. In contrast, the carbon dioxide content of blood has a nearly linear relationship to the partial pressure of carbon dioxide in the blood. As ventilation alters the partial pressure of carbon dioxide in the alveoli, so it alters the partial pressure in blood and so the carbon dioxide content of blood. Consequently, carbon dioxide removal rises and falls in proportion to ventilation and the arterial partial pressure of carbon dioxide is a good index of ventilation. Ventilation and perfusion are both less at the top of the lung than the bottom, but going up the lungs there is a greater fall in blood flow because of gravity than there is in ventilation. This means that the ratio of ventilation to perfusion is greater at the top than the bottom of the lungs. There is normally an oxygen gradient from alveolar gas to arterial blood and this gradient is widened in certain disease states, particularly those causing ventilation perfusion (V/Q) mismatch such as pulmonary embolism. Carbon dioxide binding to haemoglobin reduces its affinity for oxygen.

Respiratory • **Answers**

## 9 F,T,T,T,T

The main aspergillus related diseases are allergic asthma, allergic bronchopulmonary aspergillosis (asthmatic pulmonary eosinophilia), extrinsic allergic alveolitis, intra-cavity aspergilloma and invasive pulmonary aspergillosis. Precipitins are antibodies and can be positive in all these conditions. Skin tests are only positive in allergic asthma and allergic bronchopulmonary aspergillosis and the eosinophil count may be raised in both these conditions. Bronchiectasis can result from asthmatic pulmonary eosinophilia and pulmonary fibrosis from extrinsic allergic alveolitis.

## 10 T,T,F,T,F

The three principal congenital causes of recurrent pulmonary infection and subsequent bronchiectasis are:
- cystic fibrosis;
- hypogammaglobulinaemia and
- any form of primary ciliary dysfunction or dyskinesia such as Kartagener's syndrome.

Kartagener's syndrome consists of situs invertus, chronic sinusitis, bronchiectasis and infertility. Abnormal ciliary function reduces the normal mucociliatory clearance of infectious agents from the sinuses and chest and sperm motility is abnormal. During development, the ciliary action is abnormal resulting in a spectrum of abnormality from dextrocardia to full situs invertus. Meigs' syndrome consists of a pelvic tumour, usually ovarian and a transudative pleural effusion. Bartter's syndrome consists of hypokalaemic alkalosis, usually with high plasma renin, angiotensin II and aldosterone levels.

## 11 T,F,T,F,T

Any cause of acute extrinsic alveolitis such as Farmer's lung (a hypersensitivity reaction to micropolyspora species in

## Answers • Respiratory

mouldy hay), can result in fibrosis. Alpha-1-antitrypsin is a serine protease inhibitor (serpin) and deficiency is associated with emphysema and sometimes liver disease. Deficiency does not typically cause fibrosis. The usual genotype is known as *MM*. However, 10% of Europeans are heterozygotes for one of two variants, the *S* variant (genotype *MS*) or the Z variant (genotype *MZ*). The genotypes ZZ homozygote or *SZ* heterozygotes are associated with disease. Lung disease is principally a problem in smokers with these genotypes. Asbestos can result in:
- benign pleural plaques;
- pulmonary fibrosis with a restrictive lung defect;
- lung carcinoma and
- mesothelioma.

Ventricular septal defects can result in pulmonary hypertension, but not usually fibrosis.

## 12 T,T,F,T,F

Of the principal lung cancers, small cell lung cancer has the worst prognosis untreated and there are usually micrometastases present at presentation. For this reason chemotherapy is the treatment of choice, sometimes followed by radiotherapy. The commonest histological type of lung cancer is squamous cell carcinoma. Only a minority of patients with nonsmall cell histology, localized disease and good lung function will benefit from surgery.

## 13 T,F,T,F,F

In asbestosis, the fibrosis is predominantly in the lower and mid-zones, in sarcoidosis the mid-zones are typically the worst affected. Extrinsic allergic alveolitis usually affects the upper and mid-zones. Fibrosis associated with connective tissue disorders such as rheumatoid arthritis typically affects the lower zones.

## Respiratory • **Answers**

**14 F,T,T,T,T**

Cystic fibrosis is an autosomal recessive disorder in which the affected gene lies on the long arm of chromosome 7 and is involved in regulating transmembrane ion channel function. Both parents are usually normal because each is a carrier and the disease is recessive. Liver failure can occur leading to portal hypertension and varices. *Pseudomonas cepacia* is difficult to treat and aquisition is associated with a worsening of prognosis. Meconium ileus equivalent can occur with viscid secretions causing bowel obstruction.

**15 T,F,F,T,T**

Sarcoidosis is characterized by the presence of large numbers of activated lymphocytes in the broncho-alveolar lavage fluid. In cryptogenic fibrosing alveolitis, the predominant cell types are usually macrophages and neutrophils. Viral pneumonias are usually associated with a high broncho-alveolar lavage lymphocyte count and bacterial pneumonias with a high neutrophil count.

**16 T,T,F,T,T**

The key causes of diffuse alveolar haemorrhage throughout the lung are antibasement membrane disease (Goodpasture's disease), the systemic vasculitides (principally Wegener's granulomatosis and microscopic polyarteritis), systemic lupus erythematosus, idiopathic rapidly progressive glomerulonephritis and idiopathic pulmonary haemosiderosis. The term Cushing's syndrome is generally used to refer to any situation in which there is excess corticosteroid. Cushing's disease is the specific entity of pituitary dependent adrenal hyperplasia, which does of course result in Cushing's syndrome.

**17 T,T,F,T,F**

Pulmonary eosinophilia consists of lung shadows and a

## Answers • Respiratory

peripheral blood eosinophilia and occurs in allergic bronchopulmonary aspergillosis, drug reactions, the hypereosinophilic syndrome, the systemic vasculitides, especially Churg–Strauss syndrome and polyarteritis nodosa and parasitic infections, especially filariasis and helminth infections. In alkaptonuria there is a deficiency of homogentisic acid oxidase resulting in urine that darkens in air, black staining of cartilage and degenerative arthritis associated with this pigmentation.

### 18  T,T,F,T,F

Infection with *Chlamydia psittaci* can cause an atypical pneumonia and can be acquired from birds. Pigeon fanciers lung is caused by hypersensitivity to the birds' droppings and to the feather bloom. The pulmonary artery wedge pressure is an estimate of left atrial pressure. Lung injury can cause the so-called adult respiratory distress syndrome with fluid movement into the alveoli; however, unlike pulmonary oedema in the context of left ventricular failure, there is no requirement for a high left atrial pressure. Unlike other industrial lung diseases, beryllium characteristically can cause granuloma formation. *Legionella pneumophila* is a Gram-negative rod which is sometimes flagellated.

### 19  F,T,F,T,F

Mycoplasma species do not have a cell wall and are therefore unaffected by penicillins which inhibit cell wall synthesis. Polyclonal IgM cold agglutinins are commonly found in mycoplasma infection and may be responsible for haemolysis as they are directed against the I antigen on erythrocytes. Cryoglobulins precipitate at temperatures below 37°C, cold agglutinins are antibodies which cause more agglutination of red blood cells at 4°C than they do at 37°C. The current conventional therapy is erythromycin or tetracycline or their derivatives.

Respiratory/Rheumatology • **Answers**

## 20 F,T,T,F,T

Central sleep apnoea refers to loss of central respiratory drive resulting in periods of apnoea and hypoxia. Obstructive sleep apnoea may occur if there is upper airways obstruction during sleep. This may result from an anatomically narrowed lumen or from the loss, during rapid eye movement (REM) sleep, of the pharyngeal tone which usually keeps the airway open. In obstructive sleep apnoea, the negative pressure during inspiration can suck in and collapse the upper airways, but the positive pressure during expiration tend to open them up. Hypoxia may result in polycythaemia. Morning headaches occurring with daytime sleepiness are a characteristic symptom of sleep apnoea.

# Rheumatology

## 1 F,F,F,F,F

Rheumatoid arthritis affects women three times more frequently than men. Cerebral involvement is common in systemic lupus erythematosus, not in rheumatoid arthritis. A positive rheumatoid factor is not diagnostic in the absence of the appropriate clinical features. Although steroids can be useful, other drugs are preferred with fewer side-effects, such as methotrexate. As with other inflammatory joint disease, symptoms are typically worse after immobility such as in the morning and may be improved by movement. The opposite is typically true of mechanical injury where symptoms are made worse by movement and are worse at the end of the day.

## 2 F,F,F,F,F

Joint destruction is not usual in systemic lupus erythematosus, although it does occur. The commonest manifesta-

## Answers • Rheumatology

tions are musculoskeletal. Skin lesions are typically photosensitive and not frankly painful. Proteinuria and haematuria only occur in the presence of glomerular disease and should not be dismissed without investigation. Small joints are affected most commonly. Neuropsychiatric disease occurs in over half of patients with systemic lupus erythematosus.

### 3 F,T,F,T,F

Typically polymyalgia causes stiffness and pain in the proximal muscles, but not wasting. Polymyositis can cause wasting and pain and may be associated with skin changes (dermatomyositis) and an underlying malignancy in some cases. A proximal myopathy can occur in vitamin D deficiency.

### 4 T,F,F,T,T

The ratio of men to women with Sjögren's syndrome is 1:9. Sjögren's syndrome is a triad of dry eyes, a dry mouth and a connective tissue disease such as rheumatoid arthritis, systemic lupus erythematosus, scleroderma or mixed connective tissue disease. Schirmer's test is performed by putting a strip of filter paper under the lower eyelid. The test is abnormal if there is less than 15 mm wetting in 5 minutes. Lip biopsy is often helpful.

### 5 T,T,T,T,T

A high erythrocyte sedimentation rate can reflect either an increase in plasma viscosity due to excess globulin (antibody) formation or inflammatory activity. Often a C reactive protein (CRP) helps distinguish these causes, being raised only in the presence of inflammation, not solely in the presence of hyperviscosity.

### 6 T,T,T,F,T

The synovial fluid of an acute gouty joint if aspirated can be viscous and may have a high neutrophil count, but should be sterile on culture. Joint destruction can occur with characteristic punched out erosions. Hypertension occurs in 25–50% of patients with gout and impaired glucose tolerance and hyperlipidaemia are also associated. In the UK, 10% of patients with gout have a history of renal colic.

- The monosodium urate crystals characteristic of gout are 2–20μm long, needle shaped and negatively birefringent under polarized light.
- In contrast, the calcium pyrophosphate crystals of pseudogout are small, 1–5μm long, rod shaped positively birefringent crystals.

## 7 F,F,F,T,F

Morning stiffness should prompt a search for an underlying inflammatory condition such as ankylosing spondylitis. The erythrocyte sedimentation rate may point to infective lesions such as tuberculosis or point to myeloma or a connective tissue disorder. Tuberculosis can affect the spine and occurs in all age groups, especially in the immunocompromised or those who have lived in countries with a high prevalence of tuberculosis. Loss of the ankle reflex in the context of back pain may signify involvement of the L5 or S1 dorsal motor root. Facet joint disease typically causes pain on extension of the back. A disc prolapse can irritate the nerve root exiting from the foramina above it so that an L5–S1 disc prolapse will irritate the L5 nerve root. Any root irritation in the lower lumbar spine can cause a positive sciatic nerve stretch test. As knee extension depends principally on L3 and L4 it is not usually affected by an L5–S1 disc prolapse.

## 8 T,F,F,T,F

Antineutrophil cytoplasmic antibodies (ANCA) are frequently found in small vessel vasculitides, but are not usually present in the large vessel vasculitides such as

## Answers • Rheumatology

temporal arteritis. As the name suggests they are antibodies to cytoplasmic components in neutrophils.
- A perinuclear or pANCA is associated with microscopic polyarteritis and a cytoplasmic or cANCA with Wegener's granulomatosis.
- Typically, the antigen recognized by a pANCA is a myeloperoxidase and by a cANCA is protease 3.

### 9 F,F,F,T,T

A rheumatoid factor is an antibody which binds to IgG. Rheumatoid factors can be of IgM, IgG or rarely IgA class themselves. Antibodies are removed by plasma exchange or plasmaphaeresis but not by dialysis. Rheumatoid factors certainly occur in the absence of joint problems especially in the elderly. A number of inflammatory conditions are also associated with rheumatoid factors such as infective endocarditis.

### 10 F,F,F,T,F

Seven percent of patients with psoriasis develop arthritis which can be:
- an asymmetrical peripheral arthritis affecting the distal interphalangeal joints with a dactylitis;
- a severe deforming arthritis;
- a symmetrical small joint arthropathy like rheumatoid arthritis;
- an asymmetrical oligoarthritis often with enthesopathy including plantar fasciitis;
- ankylosing spondylitis, alone or with one of the other groups.

An enthesopathy is a disorder of a tendon insertion point. Treatment of psoriatic arthropathy is usually conservative with physical therapy and nonsteroidal anti-inflammatory drugs, but in severe cases methotrexate is of benefit.

## 11 T,T,F,T,T

Hypocomplementaemia occurs commonly in infective endocarditis, systemic lupus erythematosus and mesangio-capillary glomerulonephritis. It also occurs in essential mixed cryoglobulinaemia type II where there is an anti-IgG rheumatoid factor (an antibody to an antibody) which is itself a monoclonal IgM. Partial lipodystrophy is a condition with wasting of subcutaneous fatty tissue and is associated with type II mesangiocapillary glomerulonephritis and hypocomplementaemia.

## 12 T,T,F,T,F

Antinuclear factors are antibodies to nuclear components of cells such as DNA and are present in most patients with Sjögren's syndrome and almost all patients with systemic lupus erythematosus. There is a specific association in juvenile arthritis with iridocyclitis. Antinuclear factors are common particularly in the elderly and at low titres and are not necessarily of any significance.

## 13 T,F,T,T,T

Antiphospholipid antibodies are a family which includes antibodies to cardiolipin, antibodies which cause a positive lupus anticoagulant test and antibodies which cause a false positive VDRL test for syphilis. The characteristics of the antiphospholipid syndrome they cause are:
- thrombocytopaenia;
- spontaneous abortion;
- thrombosis and
- neurological disease.

The neurological disease may relate in part to thrombosis. Other features may include livedo reticularis. The syndrome can occur alone or in the presence of systemic lupus erythematosus.

## Answers • Rheumatology

### 14 T,T,F,T,T

In amyloidosis, there is deposition of amyloid P protein combined with another protein.

- In AL amyloid, which occurs in the presence of myeloma or other gammopathy the other protein is an antibody component derived from immunoglobulin light (L) chains.
- In AA amyloid, which occurs in the presence of persistent inflammation, the other protein is derived from an acute phase reactant serum amyloid A protein (SAA).

Amyloid deposition in the kidney can cause renal failure. A separate form of amyloid is dialysis amyloid which can occur in renal failure due to the deposition of fibrils containing beta-2-microglobulin. Beta-2-microglobulin is a component of class I major histocompatibility complex (MHC) molecules and as it is normally excreted by the kidney accumulates in patients on dialysis. Only in the case of AL amyloid is a malignancy likely, usually in the form of myeloma or lymphoma. The key to treatment is to control the underlying disease. Biopsy of any affected tissue can be diagnostic. Traditionally, rectal biopsy was used to make the diagnosis, but rectal biopsy is not always positive. Mortality can be significant, especially in the presence of cardiac involvement. Serum amyloid P can be radio-labelled and the deposition of this used in a radio-isotope scan to detect sites of amyloid deposition. Treatment of familial Mediterranean fever with colchicine reduces the incidence of amyloid deposition.

### 15 F,F,F,F,T

The principal seronegative arthritides are:
- ankylosing spondylitis;
- psoriatic arthritis;
- reactive arthritis and
- arthritis associated with inflammatory bowel disease.

## Rheumatology • **Answers**

The major HLA association is with HLA-B27 and ankylosing spondylitis, though the prevalence of B27 is also increased in patients with the other seronegative arthritides who develop spinal involvement. Reactive arthritis is typically triggered by a sexually transmitted disease, especially chlamydial urethritis or bowel infection by organisms such as *Shigella*, *Salmonella* and *Yersinia*. By definition, rheumatoid factor is absent in the seronegative arthritides. Iritis can occur in ankylosing spondylitis, reactive arthritis and inflammatory bowel disease.

## 16 F,F,F,T,F

Penicillamine can cause proteinuria and membranous nephropathy, as can gold, given orally or injected. Membranous nephropathy can cause nephrotic syndrome. Methotrexate is monitored by regular liver function tests. Cyclophosphamide can be helpful if the disease develops into frank vasculitis. Steroids at a low dose such as 2.5–5mg per day of prednisolone can be useful, but if possible a steroid sparing agent such as methotrexate should be used. Cyclosporin is of benefit, in some cases, but requires careful monitoring of renal function.

## 17 T,F,F,F,T

Ibuprofen is less likely to cause renal complications than diclofenac, indomethacin or piroxicam. Many topical preparations are absorbed and there are reports of renal disease caused by topical nonsteroidal anti-inflammatories. Risk factors for renal complications are well recognized and include:
- advanced age;
- male sex;
- dehydration;
- congestive heart disease and
- pre-existing renal disease.

## Answers • Rheumatology

Phenylbutazone is particularly useful in ankylosing spondylitis, but requires haematological monitoring because of the risk of aplastic anaemia.

### 18 F,F,T,T,F

In Paget's disease of bone the key problem appears to be excessive osteoclast activity with bone destruction and the production of new bone which is highly vascularized. Calcium and phosphate are normal, alkaline phosphatase is usually raised and urine hydroxy-proline excretion is raised. Calcitonin derivatives and etidronate can be helpful. Bony enlargement of the pituitary fossa can cause diabetes insipidus. Sarcomatous change occurs but is rare.

### 19 F,T,F,F,F

There is a reduction in bone matrix (osteoid) in osteoporosis. Withdrawal of sex hormones after the menopause is the main cause in women, but osteoporsis can also occur in men, especially the elderly or those such as men with Klinefelter's syndrome who have sex hormone deficiency. In Klinefelter's syndrome, the karyotype is XXY and there is usually testicular atrophy, gynaecomastia and infertility. Bone densitometry is the best method of routine assessment and is a measure of the penetrance of X-rays through the bone at defined anatomical points. Serum calcium, phosphate and alkaline phosphatase are usually normal. Etidronate and hormone replacement therapy can both improve bone density.

### 20 T,F,T,F,F

Osteomalacia is the result of inadequate mineralization of a normal bone matrix (osteoid). Causes include renal disease, dietary insufficiency of vitamin D and malabsorption. A proximal myopathy can occur making standing up from a sitting position difficult. The kidney contains a 1-alpha-hydroxylase which converts 25-hydroxycholecalciferol to 1, 25-dihydroxycholecalciferol. In renal disease this activity is diminished so treatment is with 1-alpha-hydroxycholecalciferol to bypass the renal step. Typically, calcium and phosphate may be low and alkaline phosphatase elevated. Renal insufficiency may tend to increase the phosphate level. Bone biopsy is not normally necessary, but is often diagnostic.

# Mathematical medicine

### 1 F,F,F,F,F

Various measures can be used to describe the distribution of data, but in simple cases, two types of statistic are used. Usually, the first statistic defines a central value such as the arithmetic mean about which the data is spread. The second statistic generally defines the extent to which the data spread or deviate about this point, and often the standard deviation is the statistic used for this purpose. Statistics defining a central point include the arithmetic mean, the median and the mode as illustrated in Fig. 11.

- Usually the arithmetical mean is used and this is the sum of the values of the data divided by the number of observations. In this case the arithmetical mean is 4 mM as the sum of the serum potassium values is 36 and this is divided by 9 because there are nine observations.
- The mode is simply the most frequently occurring value which is 3 mM.
- The median is the point which lies midway between the two extreme values when the observations are ranked in order. In this case there are nine values so the median is the value of the fifth observation when ranked in order which is 3.5 mM

## Answers • Mathematical medicine

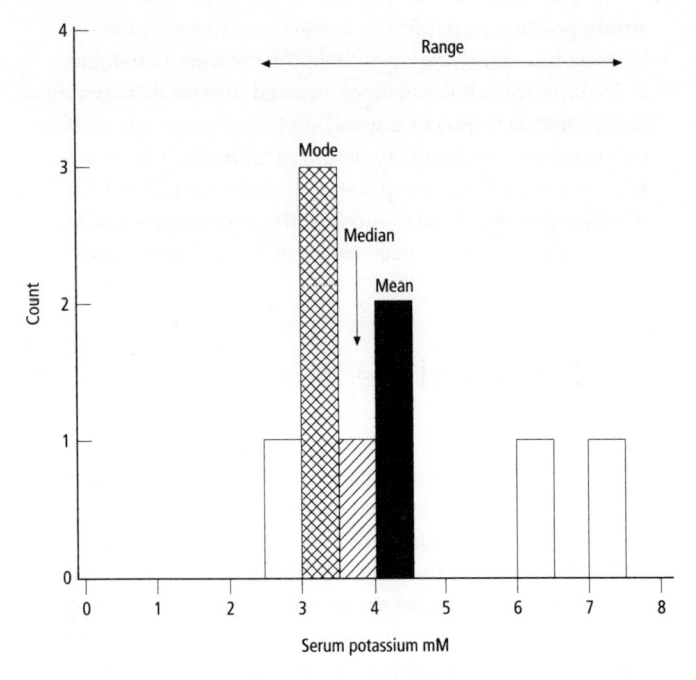

**Figure 11** A histogram illustrating the frequency of serum potassium values in the small sample of patients.

| Rank order | 1 | 2 | 3 | 4 | 5 | 6 | 7 | 8 | 9 |
|---|---|---|---|---|---|---|---|---|---|
| Serum potassium | 2.5 | 3 | 3 | 3 | 3.5 | 4 | 4 | 6 | 7 |

The standard deviation is a measure of the extent to which the data which conforms to the normal distribution is spread about the arithmetic mean. It is calculated by working out the extent to which each point differs from the mean and using this information to compute an average deviation from that mean. The way in which it is calculated is discussed below. However, even the most extreme points (2.5 mM and 7 mM) on this distribution of potassium values are less than 5 mM different from the arithmetic mean of 4, so the standard deviation must be less than 5 mM. The range of the data is the difference between the highest and the lowest values, in this case the range is $7 - 2.5 = 4.5$.

## 2 F,T,F,F,F

The standard deviation is a measure of the spread or dispersion of data about the mean and is computed as follows. In the first place, the arithmetic mean (m) is calculated, which in the example in question 1 is $36 \div 9 = 4$. For each sample value, the difference between the sample value and the mean is computed and this value is squared so that all such values are positive. All these squared differences from the mean are added together and their sum is divided by $(n-1)$ where $n$ is the number of observations to give the average squared difference from the mean. $n-1$ is used rather than $n$ because this gives the distribution about the sample mean and provides a better estimate of the population mean. This value is now known as the sample variance. However, this is the average squared difference from the mean and to compute the average unsquared difference from the mean, the positive square root of the variance is calculated and is the standard deviation.

Mean serum potassium = 4
Number of observations $n = 9$

| Serum potassium | 2.5 | 3 | 3 | 3 | 3.5 | 4 | 4 | 6 | 7 |
|---|---|---|---|---|---|---|---|---|---|
| Difference from mean | -1.5 | -1 | -1 | -1 | -0.5 | 0 | 0 | 2 | 3 |
| Squared difference from mean | 2.25 | 1 | 1 | 1 | 0.25 | 0 | 0 | 4 | 9 |

Sum of squared differences = 18.5
Variance 18.5/8 = 2.3125
Standard deviation = $\sqrt{}$ variance
= $\sqrt{}$ 2.3125 = 1.52

### Answers • Mathematical medicine

In summary, the formula for the standard deviation is:
Standard deviation (SD) =

$$\sqrt{\frac{\sum_{i=1}^{n}(x_i-\bar{x})^2}{n-1}}$$

which can be rewritten as:

$$\sqrt{\frac{\sum x^2 - \frac{(\sum x)^2}{n}}{n-1}}$$

where:
  $\bar{x}$ is the mean
  $x_i$ is the value of the $i$ th sample
  $n$ is the number of observations

and

$$\sum_{i=1}^{n} x_i$$

stands for the sum of all values of $x$ from $i = 1$ to $i = n$ and is usually shortened to

$$\sum x.$$

If the data follows a normal distribution then:
• approximately 68% of the values lie within one standard deviation of the mean;
• approximately 95% of the values lie within two standard deviations of the mean and
• approximately 99.7% of the values lie within three standard deviations of the mean.

The standard deviation alone only provides information about the spread of data about the mean and not about the mean itself. As the dispersion or spread of the data gets greater, so the standard deviation gets greater.

Mathematical medicine • **Answers**

This question also highlights the difference between the population and the sample.
- The sample refers to the observations which have actually been made and the mean and standard deviation of the sample can be precisely calculated as shown above.
- The population refers to the entire group from which the sample was drawn and the mean and standard deviation can only be estimated from the sample values.

The set of serum potassium values 2.5, 3, 3, 3, 3.5, 4, 4, 6 and 7 might have been taken from nine random patients with diabetes and forms a sample of the total population of patients with diabetes. Although we do not know the mean value of serum potassium in the total population of diabetic patients, our sample enables us to estimate this value by calculating the sample mean which is 4.

## 3 T,F,T,F,T

It is useful to know how reliable sample statistics such as the sample mean and standard deviation are as estimates of the true population values and the standard error of the mean (SEM) and confidence intervals or limits are used for this purpose.
- The standard error of the mean is calculated by dividing the standard deviation (SD) of the sample data by the square root of the number of observations ($n$). As the standard error of the mean gets bigger, so the range within which the population mean can be expected to lie gets wider and estimates of the population mean become less accurate. The lower the standard deviation and the higher the number of observations in the sample, then the lower will be the SEM and the more accurate the prediction of the population mean. The standard error of the mean is inversely proportional to the square root of the sample size and proportional to the standard deviation.
- $SEM = SD/\sqrt{n}$;

- Confidence limits allow the prediction of the population mean with a precise probability. The 95% confidence limits enclose a range within which the population mean can be expected to lie in 95% of cases (or 19 times out of 20) and is calculated by the formula:

   95% confidence limits = sample mean + or − $t$(SEM)

   where $t$ is Students $t$ statistic which is obtained by consulting statistical tables.

## 4 F,T,F,T,T

It is often necessary to determine whether two sets of data are different or similar. For example, in a comparison of two antihypertensive drugs it is useful to compare systolic blood pressures in the two groups to see if they differ significantly. Parametric data conforms to a mathematically defined distribution such as the normal or binomial distribution. The normal distribution can be completely described by its mean and standard deviation and is symmetrical about the mean.

- Students $t$ test is used to assess whether the sample means are significantly different. It is suitable for parametric data and assumes that the variances of the two samples are the same.
- The $F$ test compares the ratio of these two sample variances to see whether the two samples come from populations with the same variance and so whether they are suitable for the $t$ test.

Kaplan–Meier analysis is used to examine the probability of survival with time such as prognosis with time after a diagnosis of cancer.

## 5 F,F,T,F,F

Risk factors for a given disease can be evaluated prospectively or retrospectively. It is usual to calculate the relative risk in a retrospective study and the odds ratio in a prospective study. Confidence intervals can be calculated for both relative risks and odds ratios.

• In prospective studies, relative risk can be calculated by following groups which differ for the risk factor and observing the number that develop the disease. If 8 out of 100 smokers and 4 out of 100 nonsmokers get coronary heart disease then the relative risk for heart disease in smokers is $(8/100)/(4/100) = 2$.

• In a retrospective case control study, it is possible to take a group of people with the disease and compare these to carefully matched controls without the disease. If 70 out of 100 patients with heart disease are smokers then the odds of a patient being a smoker are $70:(100-70)$ or $7:3$. If only 40 out of 100 patients in the control group are smokers then the odds of being a smoker are $4:6$. The odds ratio is then $(7/3):(4/6) = 3.5$ which tells us that patients are 3.5 times more likely than controls to be smokers. The higher the odds ratio, the higher the implied risk, if other risk factors are controlled for and the study is not flawed.

6 **T,T,T,F,T**

Both correlation and regression can be used to characterize a relationship between two variables such as weight and blood pressure, but they do this in different ways:

• correlation describes the strength of the association;

• regression analysis describes the mathematical equation which links the two variables, regardless of how good the association is.

A correlation coefficient can be calculated using Pearson's method or a rank correlation method such as Kendall's or Spearman's. The correlation coefficient ($r$) varies from $-1$ to $+1$, with 0 being no correlation, $+1$ a positive straight line relationship between the two variables and $-1$ a negative straight line relationship. Regression analysis will provide an equation which links two variables $x$ and $y$. Linear regression will provide the best straight line equation of the form $y = ax + b$ linking the two variables where a is the slope of the graph and b is the intercept of the line on the y axis. However, linear regression does not directly measure the strength of the association in the way that correlation does.

7 T,F,T,F,T

Multiple regression analysis provides a means of determining the extent to which various variables such as age, weight and blood pressure each contribute to a variable such as the incidence of heart disease. Probabilities are usually measured from 0 to 1. The $p$ value quoted for a result is the probability that the result has occurred by chance. A $p$ value of 0.05 means that there is a 5% or 1 in 20 probability that the result occurs by chance and this 5% level is conventionally used as the threshold for significance.

Chi square analysis can be used on categorical data such as a group comparison between survival from meningitis in boys and girls. A table is usually constructed as shown:

*Observed values*

|        | Dead | Survived | Total |
|--------|------|----------|-------|
| Male   | 44   | 56       | 100   |
| Female | 56   | 44       | 100   |
| Total  | 100  | 100      |       |

*Expected values*

|        | Dead | Survived | Total |
|--------|------|----------|-------|
| Male   | 50   | 50       | 100   |
| Female | 50   | 50       | 100   |
| Total  | 100  | 100      |       |

Chi square analysis compares the observed numbers in the different categories with the expected numbers if the groups were distributed by chance. This allows the calculation of the probability that the difference in the distribution between the different categories occurs by chance. If the number in any category is small (<5) then Fisher's exact test must be applied.

In the evaluation of any relationship between non-categorical data, a scattergram should be inspected to visualize the relationship and to check the distribution of the data. The Mann–Whitney $U$ test or Mann–Whitney–Wilcoxon test can be used in place of the Students $t$ test when comparing two independent groups of data which are non-parametric.

## 8 F,T,T,F,T

The power of the study is the probability that the study will detect a difference of a given degree in the incidence of thrombosis between the groups studied, with a defined statistical significance. For example, the study could have an 80% probability of detecting a 15% difference in the incidence of thrombosis with the result being significant at the 5% level ($p$ for the study being ≤0.05). The greater the sample size, the greater the power of the study and the greater the probability that a true difference between the groups will be detected. If the study group is at high risk of venous thrombosis, such as a population of elderly patients following hip surgery, then the number of thromboses should be high and thus the power of the study to detect a reduction in this should be higher than in a low risk population such as young male adults undergoing tooth extraction.

Case control studies are generally retrospective studies to compare risk factors for a condition. A randomized controlled trial is ideal for this type of study. Patients are admitted to the study if they fulfil certain entry criteria which determine that they are a uniform population, and are then randomized to placebo or drug therapy. Retrospective analysis can be informative, but is not always reasonable. If, for example, 20 variables were examined at the 5% ($p \leq 0.05$)

### Answers • Mathematical medicine

significance level to see if they predicted a good outcome from prophylaxis then one would expect to show an association with one variable by chance, because that is what the 5% probability predicts; (5 in 100 = 1 in 20). The calculation of the power of a study is complex, but a pilot study will provide estimates of the parameters that determine power.

### 9 T,T,F,F,T

The table shows the possible results for a diagnostic test of this type.

|  | Infected | Uninfected | Total |
|---|---|---|---|
| Test result positive | a | b | a+b |
| Test result negative | c | d | c+d |
| Total | a+c | b+d | n |

Sensitivity = $a/(a+c)$
Specificity = $d/(b+d)$
Positive predictive value = $a/(a+b)$
Negative predictive value = $d/(c+d)$

Sensitivity and specificity define the probability of the disease state being correctly identified. The denominator is always the disease group and the numerator is always a test result.
• The sensitivity is the number of correctly identified true positives or truly infected people with a positive test result.
• The specificity is the number of correctly identified true negatives or truly uninfected people with a negative test result.

Predictive values define the probability of the test result being correct in the population studied. The denominator is always the test result and the numerator the disease state.
• The positive predictive value is the number of people with a positive test result who have infection.

- The negative predictive value is the number of people with a negative test result who are uninfected.

The prevalence in the study is $a+c/n$ and the predictive values only hold for a population with this prevalence. Baye's theorem allows the calculation of test results for other populations with a different known prevalence given the values of sensitivity and specificity, which do not vary from population to population. Baye's theorem states that the positive predictive value for the new population, i.e. the probability of disease when the test result is positive is equal to

= (sensitivity × prevalence)/((sensitivity × prevalence) + ((1 − specificity) × (1 − prevalence)))

The likelihood ratio is the ratio of the sensitivity to the specificity and this is equivalent to the probability of getting a positive test result if the patient is infected. The more sensitive the test, the higher the likelihood ratio:

likelihood ratio = sensitivity/specificity
= probability of a positive test in an infected patient/
(1 − probability of a positive result in an uninfected patient).

**10 T,F,T,T,F**

In any follow up study, it is useful to be able to predict the probability that a patient with a given disease will be alive at certain times after diagnosis. The crudest way of doing this is simply to look at the proportion or percentage of the initial group still alive at a fixed time. If, for example, 27% of patients are alive at 5 years then the 5 year survival is 27%. However, it is also very instructive to have a continuous survival curve over the entire study period as this allows the prediction of survival at any time interval and may reveal patterns such as a sudden fall in survival after diagnosis or a plateau after a given time period. Such a survival probability

## Answers • Mathematical medicine

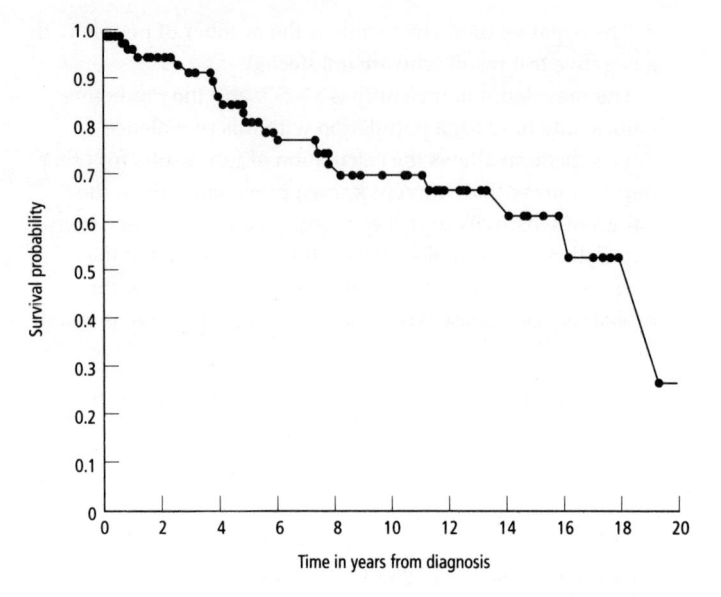

**Figure 12** A Kaplan–Meier survival curve for patients with a slowly progressing disease. Survival falls with time and each point represents the outcome of a single patient. Where the slope falls, the end point was death, where the slope is horizontal, the patient was lost to follow-up.

curve can be calculated by Kaplan–Meier survival analysis, an example of which is shown in Fig. 12.

In principle this kind of analysis works out the probability of death in the time interval between each observation. Taking the moment of diagnosis as time zero, the patients are ranked in order according to the length of follow up. End points are death or loss from the study for other reasons, usually loss to follow-up in a clinic. If the event is a death then the probability of death in the period since the previous patients end point is $1/n$ where $n$ is the number of patients still alive and the probability of survival is $1 - (1/n)$. This survival probability is then multiplied by the cumulative probability of survival up until that point to produce a new cumulative survival probability. If the event is not a death then the probability of survival is not changed from the value for the preceding time period. As the number of patients followed up decreases with time, the confidence limits for the survival probability get broader.

| Patient | Length of follow-up | End point | Survival probability | Number in study |
|---|---|---|---|---|
| 1 | 1 year | Death | $(1-1/10) = 0.9$ | 10 |
| 2 | 2 years | Death | $(1-1/9) \times 0.9 = 0.8$ | 9 |
| 3 | 3 years | Lost to follow-up | $(1) \times 0.9 = 0.8$ | 8 |
| 4 | 4 years | Death | $(1-1/7) \times 0.8 = 0.69$ | 7 |

Cox's method is also known as proportional hazards regression analysis and is a method for producing an equation which predicts survival on the basis of a number of variables such as age, etc.

# Index

*Note*: page numbers in *italic* refer to figures.

A antigen antibodies 34, 113–14
ABO incompatibility 34, 114
acarbose 88
acetylcholine 135, 136
achalasia 101
acromegaly 85, 87
action potential, cardiac 16, 73–4
acute tubular necrosis 87
acyclovir 42, 51, 129, 152
Addison's disease 84
adenosine 49, 80, 148
adrenal hyperplasia, congenital 83
adrenaline 19, 51, 82, 152
  renal effects 41, 127
adrenergic receptors 82
adrenocorticotrophic hormone (ACTH) 89
adriamycin 51, 150
adult respiratory distress syndrome 57, 164
air embolism 52, 153
airway obstruction 53, 157
alcohol abuse 102, 105
aldosterone 83, 130
alkalosis, hypochloraemic 101–2
alkaptonuria 57, 102, 164
allopurinol 40, 50, 124, 150
all-trans retinoic acid 34, 113
alpha-1-antitrypsin deficiency 56, 162
5-alpha-reductase 83, *84*
  deficiency 83
Alport's disease 134
alveolar haemorrhage, diffuse 57, 133–4, 163
alveolitis
  cryptogenic fibrosing 57, 163
  extrinsic allergic 55, 56, 57, 161, 162, 163
aminoglutethimide 53, 156
aminoglycosides 125
aminophylline 49, 52, 148, 155
amiodarone 53, 155
amitriptyline overdose 53, 157
amoebic disease 38, 121
amphotericin 42, 129
ampicillin 51, 152
amplification refractory mutation system-polymerase chain reaction (ARMS-PCR) 132–3
amyloidosis 61, 170
  in Creutzfeldt–Jakob disease 44, 137
  peripheral neuropathy 138, 140
  in renal failure 43, 61, 133, 170
anaemia 33, 112–13
  aplastic 33, 107
  megaloblastic 30, 44, 104–5, 136
  microcytic 32, 110
  pernicious 104
  sideroblastic 110
*Ancylostoma duodenale* 121–2
androgens 83, 87
  excess 86
angiotensin converting enzyme inhibitors
  in diabetic nephropathy 88, 128–9
  in hypertension 51, 151

# Index

angiotensin converting enzyme inhibitors *(Cont.)*
  in renal artery stenosis 40, 125–6
  *see also* captopril
ankylosing spondylitis 170–1
  aortic regurgitation 79, 80
  respiratory problems 54, 56, 159, 162
anterior cerebral artery occlusion 48, 144, 146
antiarrhythmics, class 4, 81–2
antidiuretic hormone, syndrome of inappropriate secretion (SIADH) 87, 156
antigenic drift 119
antigenic shift 119
antihypertensive therapy 51, 151
antimitochondrial antibodies 100
antineutrophil cytoplasmic antibodies 60, 167–8
antinuclear antibodies 60–1, 169
antiphospholipid antibodies 61, 169
antiphospholipid syndrome 45, 105, 137, 169
antithrombin III deficiency 109
antituberculous therapy 38, 122
aorta
  coarctation 79
  dissection of thoracic 18, 79
aortic stenosis 15, 16, 19, 70, 82–3
aortic valve
  biscuspid 82
  regurgitation 18, 80
arthritis
  inflammatory bowel disease 98, 170
  juvenile 60, 169
  psoriatic 60, 168, 170
  reactive 28, 99, 170–1
  rheumatoid *see* rheumatoid arthritis
asbestosis/asbestos exposure 56, 162
*Ascaris lumbricoides* 38, 121

ascites 27, 98
aspergillosis, allergic bronchopulmonary 57, 161, 164
aspergillus related diseases 55, 161
aspirin 16–17, 74–5
  in gout 50, 149
  in myocardial infarction prevention 51, 74–5, 151
  overdose 53, 156–7
  platelet actions 50, 74, 149
  in stroke prevention 44, 136
asthma 54, 101, 158
  adenosine in 49, 148
  aspergillus related 55, 161
  atenolol in 52, 154
  hypoxia in 54, 159
  respiratory function testing 53, 157
atenolol 51, 52, 152, 154
atrial fibrillation 81, 82
  stroke prevention 44, 136
atrial septal defect (ASD) 16, 72–3
atrioventricular block 82
atropine 25, 52, 94, 152
autonomic neuropathy, diabetic 24, 92, 101
azathioprine 53, 157

back pain 59, 167
bacterial infections 38, 113–4, 122–3
  *see* individual organisms
B antigen antibodies 34, 113–14
Barrett's oesophagus 101
Bartter's syndrome 55, 102, 161
basilar artery 43, 134, *135*
B cell development 33, 112
BCG vaccination 35, 115
Behçet's disease 27, 99
benzodiazepines 52, 152
beryllium exposure 57, 164
beta blockers 77, 91, 98, 151, 152
beta-2 microglobulin 170

# Index

biguanides 88
bilharzia *see* schistosomiasis
bleomycin 51, 150
blood
   cell development 33, 112
   crossmatching 34, 114
   transfusion 34, 113–14
bone marrow transplantation 109
books 8, 10–11
*Borrelia burgdorferi* infection (Lyme disease) 35, 47, 116, 142
bradycardia 19, 81
brain, blood supply 134, *135*
brainstem damage 47–8, 143–4
breastfeeding, antihypertensive therapy 51, 151
bromocriptine 87
bronchiectasis 55, 161
broncho-alveolar lavage, lymphocyte counts 57, 163
Budd–Chiari syndrome 27, 98
bumetanide 52, 155

calcium channel blockers 148, 151
calcium ions, in cardiac action potential 16, 74
campylobacter infections 28, 99
cancer chemotherapy 51, 150
*Candida albicans* infections 37, 120–1
Caplan's syndrome 54, 159
captopril
   in renal artery stenosis 40, 125–6
   renal blood flow effects 41, 127
carbamazepine 53, 156
carbimazole 85
carbon dioxide
   excretion 55, 160
   haemoglobin binding 55, 160
carcinoid syndrome 28, 100
cardiac action potential 16, 73–4

cardiac cycle 15, 69
cardiology 15–18, 69–83
carotid pulse, dicrotic notch 15, 69
carotid stenosis, severe 44, 136
carpal tunnel syndrome 85
case-control studies 64, 65, 179, 181
catecholamines 19, 52, 82, 154
cavernous sinus 44, 134
ceramics industry 54, 159
cerebral oedema 102
cerebrospinal fluid
   lymphocytes/monocytes 48, 144
   protein content 48, 144
Chagas' disease 75–6, 101
Charcot–Marie–Tooth disease 46, 47, 139–40, 142
Chi square analysis 65, 180–1
*Chlamydia psittaci* 119, 164
*Chlamydia trachomatis* 37, 119
chloroquine 35, 116
chlorpromazine 51, 152
chlorpropamide 50, 53, 149, 156
cholangitis, primary sclerosing 28, 100
cholesterol
   HDL 76
   serum total 76
   in steroid biosynthesis 83, *84*
Churg–Strauss syndrome 60, 158, 167
chylomicrons 153
cimetidine 40, 124
ciprofloxacin 51, 151
cirrhosis 27, 98
   primary biliary 98, 100
cisplatin 51, 150
clotting, blood 33, 111–12
coal miners 54, 159
cocaine 48, 49, 144, 147–8
coeliac disease 34, 104–5, 113
colchicine 50, 149–50
cold agglutinins 107, 164
confidence limits 63, 177, 178, 179

# Index

congenital adrenal hyperplasia 83
Congo red stain 54, 158
corneal reflex 48, 143–4
coronary artery disease 17, 76–7
correlation
　analysis 64, 179
　coefficient 64, 179
corticosteroids 23, 89–91
　excess 86, 90, 163
　in rheumatoid arthritis 61, 171
corticotrophin releasing factor (CRF) 89
cortisol 83, 90–1
co-trimoxazole 51, 151
Cox's proportional hazards analysis 66, 185
C reactive protein (CRP) 110, 166
creatinine 39, 124
Creutzfeldt–Jakob disease 44, 137
Crohn's disease 27, 98
crossmatching, blood 34, 114
cryoglobins 99, 107, 164
cryoglobulinaemia 27, 99
　essential mixed 59, 60, 166, 169
cryptococcal infection 118, 144
cryptosporidium 28, 99, 118
Cushing's disease 90, 163
Cushing's syndrome (excess corticosteroids) 57, 86, 90, 163
cyanosis, in neonates 16, 72–3
cyclophosphamide 51, 61, 150, 171
cyclosporin 39, 40, 124, 125, 171
cysticercosis 123
cystic fibrosis 55, 56, 101, 102, 161, 163
cytomegalovirus infections 37, 57, 119, 163
cytotoxic drugs 50–1, 150

dexamethasone suppression test 91

diabetes insipidus 62, 87, 172
diabetes mellitus
　antihypertensive therapy 51, 151
　*Candida albicans* infections 121
　insulin dependent 22, 87–8
　noninsulin dependent 22, 88
　treatment 50, 149
diabetic autonomic neuropathy 24, 92, 101
diabetic nephropathy 41–2, 88, 128–9
diabetic neuropathy 88, 140
diabetic retinopathy 88
diarrhoea 26, 97
　traveller's 51, 151
digoxin 75, 81–2
　overdose 53, 157
diltiazem 79
2,3-diphosphoglycerate (2,3-DPG) 31, 108
diphtheria 38, 46, 123, 139, 140
disc prolapse 59, 167
diuretics, thiazide 50, 51, 150, 151
dobutamine 19, 82, 154
doll's eye reflex 47–8, 143
dopamine
　adrenaline and 51, 152
　inotropic action 19, 82
　mechanism of action 52, 154
　in Parkinson's disease 46, 141
　renal blood flow effects 41, 127
　in renal failure 40, 124
drugs
　anti-hypertensives in pregnancy and breastfeeding 51, 151
　combinations 51, 151–2
　in glucose-6-phosphate dehydrogenase deficiency 32, 110
　hypokalaemia and 52, 155
　hyponatraemia and 53, 156
　interacting with warfarin 30, 105

# Index

mechanisms of action 51–2, 152
nephrotoxic 40, 124–5
in porphyria 104
renal blood flow and 41, 127
renal excretion 39–40, 124
skin reactions 53, 155–6
Duchenne muscular dystrophy 47, 86, 142
ductus arteriosus, patent 15, 16, 70–1, 72
duodenal ulceration 93
dysphagia 28, 101
dysphasia
expressive 48, 144–6
receptive 144–6
dystrophia myotonica 47, 86, 142–3

Ebstein's anomaly 16, 72–3
*Echinococcus* 123
edrophonium bromide 46, 140
Ehlers–Danlos syndrome 112–13
electrocardiograph (ECG)
capture beats 80
fusion beats 80
left axis deviation 80
potassium-associated changes 15–16, 71
QTc interval 15, 69–70
right axis deviation 18–19, 80
ELISA 94–5
emergencies, medical 3
emphysema 53, 157–8
endocarditis, infective 60, 80, 168, 169
endocrinology 20–4, 83–93
endoscopic retrograde cholangio-pancreatogram (ERCP) 100
*Entamoeba histolytica* 121
*Enterobius vermicularis* 38, 121
Epstein–Barr virus 37, 119
erythema
chronicum migrans 116
multiforme 53, 155
nodosum 53, 156
toxic 53, 155
erythrocyte sedimentation rate (ESR) 59, 166
erythropoietin 133
ethambutol 38, 122
examination
past papers 8
preparation
general 1–5
practical revision 9–11
specific 6–8
questions *see* questions, exam
technique 11–12

facet joint disease 59, 167
factor V Leiden 109
Fallot's tetralogy 54, 159
familial mediterranean fever 61, 170
farmer's lung 56, 161–2
ferritin, serum 110
filariasis 57, 164
finasteride 83
Fisher's exact test 181
fluconazole 124
fludrocortisone 53, 156
fluoxetine 47, 49, 141, 147
fluvoxamine 49, 141, 147
folate deficiency 104–5
follicle stimulating hormone 92
Friedreich's ataxia 45, 139
frusemide 51, 53, 151–2, 156
*F* test 64, 178
fungal infections 37, 120–1

galactorrhoea 22, 87
gallstones, impacted 94
ganciclovir 39, 123
gastric acid secretion 25, 94
gastric adenocarcinoma 93
gastric mucosa associated lymphoid tissue (MALT) lymphoma 93
gastric ulceration 93
gastrin 25, 94

# Index

gastritis, antral 93
gastroenterology 25–9, 93–104
gastrointestinal infections 28, 99–100
Gaucher's disease 81
gene sequencing 133
giardiasis (*Giardia lamblia*) 28, 99–100
globin genes 31, 108
glomerular sclerosis, focal segmental 41, 128
glomerulonephritis
  focal segmental glomerular sclerosis 41, 128
  idiopathic rapidly progressive 57, 163
  Goodpastures syndrome 43, 53, 133–4, 157
  IgA nephropathy 41, 127
  minimal change nephropathy 41, 128
  membranous nephropathy 40–41, 127
  mesangiocapillary 60, 169
glucagon 25, 94
glucose-6-phosphate dehydrogenase deficiency (G-6-PD) 32, 110
glutathione 52, 154–5
glycogen storage diseases 84
goitre, toxic nodular 85
gold therapy 42, 53, 61, 129, 156, 171
Goodpasture's syndrome 43, 53, 133–4, 157
gout 50, 59, 149–50, 166–7
granulocyte–macrophage colony stimulating factor (GM-CSF) 33, 112
Graves disease 85
growth hormone 20, 85, 86
Guillain–Barré syndrome 46, 140

haematology 30–4, 104–14
haemoglobin 31, 108
  carbon dioxide binding 55, 160
  low 33, 112–13
haemoglobinuria, paroxysmal nocturnal 31, 107
haemolytic uraemic syndrome 105
haemophilia 111
haemoptysis 75
haem synthesis *103*
halofantrine 35, 116–17
HDL cholesterol 76
headache, in sleep apnoea 58, 165
Heaf test 54, 158
heart block 77, 81
heart failure, congestive 17, 75–6
heart rate, slow 19, 81
heart sounds
  second 15, 70–1
  third 15, 69
*Helicobacter pylori* 25, 26, 93, 97
heparin 86, 105
hepatic encephalopathy 102
hepatitis
  chronic active 98
  chronic persistent 98
  viral causes 37, 119
hepatitis B virus infection 102
hepatitis C virus infection 26, 27, 94–5, 99, 102
hepatocellular carcinoma (hepatoma) 27, 98
hepatomegaly *see* liver, enlarged
hereditary motor and sensory neuropathy (Charcot–Marie–Tooth disease) 46, 47, 139–40, 142
HIV infection *see* human immunodeficiency virus (HIV) infection
HLA-B27 171
Hodgkin's disease 34, 113
homocystinuria 79
hookworms 38, 110, 121–2
hormone replacement therapy, post menopausal 23, 91
human immunodeficiency virus (HIV) infection 28, 36, 39, 99, 117–18, 123

# Index

Huntington's disease 47, 143
hydatid disease 39, 123
hydralazine 42, 124, 129
5-hydroxy indoleacetic acid (5-HIAA) 91, 100
21 hydroxylase deficiency 83
5-hydroxytryptamine (5-HT; serotonin) 47, 49, 141, 147
hypercalcaemia 87, 89, 131
hypercholesterolaemia, familial 153
hyperkalaemia
  ECG changes 15–16, 71
  in renal tubular acidosis 130
hyperlipidaemias 153–4
hyperlipoproteinaemia, remnant 154
hyperparathyroidism
  nephrocalcinosis in 42, 131
  primary 89
  in renal failure 43, 89, 133
  secondary 89, 133
  tertiary 89, 133
hyperprolactinaemia 87, 93
hypertension 42, 79, 129
  in diabetic nephropathy 129
  drug therapy 51, 151
  gout and 59, 167
  systolic, as stroke risk factor 44, 136
hyperthyroidism (thyrotoxicosis) 20–1, 85, 86
hypertriglyceridaemia, familial 154
hyperviscosity syndrome 33, 111
hypocalcaemia
  ECG effects 15, 70
  in malabsorption 93
hypocomplementaemia 60, 169
hypogammaglobulinaemia 55, 97, 161
hypoglycaemia 20, 84, 88, 102
  in falciparum malaria 120
  in total parenteral nutrition 153

hypogonadism 86
hypokalaemia
  drugs causing 52, 155
  ECG changes 15–16, 71
  in hypochloraemic alkalosis 102
  in renal tubular acidosis 130
hyponatraemia, drugs causing 53, 156
hypophosphataemia 52, 153
hyposplenism 106
hypothyroidism 81
hypoxia 54, 159

ibuprofen 171
IgA nephropathy 41, 127
index cards 9–10
indomethacin 40, 41, 124–5, 127
infections 34–9, 114–23
  gastrointestinal 28, 99–100
  urinary tract 40, 125
infertility 24, 92–3
inflammatory bowel disease 27, 98, 170
influenza virus infection 36, 118–19
insulin stress test 91
interleukin-6 112
internal capsule lesions 48, 146
intracranial pressure, raised 81
intrinsic factor 104
iridocyclitis 60, 169
iritis 61, 62
iron deficiency 110
irritable bowel syndrome (IBS) 26–7, 97
isoniazid 38, 51, 122, 151
isoprenaline 19, 52, 82, 154

jaundice 27, 37, 98, 119
Jervell–Lange–Nielsen syndrome 70
journals, medical 2–3
jugular venous pressure (JVP) 16, 71

# Index

jugular venous pulse (JVP) 15, 69
  cannon waves 79–80
kala azar 36, 117
Kaplan–Meier survival analysis 64, 66, 178, 183–5
Kartagener's syndrome 55, 161
kidney
  drug elimination 39, 124
  medullary sponge 131
  polycystic disease 43, 131–3
  transplantation 129
Klinefelter's syndrome 62, 92–3, 172
kuru 44, 137
Kussmaul's sign 69, 71

labetalol 51, 151
lactose intolerance 97
lactulose 97, 102
larva migrans
  cutaneous 122
  visceral 117
L-dopa 51, 152
lead toxicity 104, 140
left ventricular end diastolic pressure 76
*Legionella pneumophila* 57, 164
leishmaniasis 36, 107, 117
leprosy 35, 46, 115, 138, 139, 140
leukaemia 144
  acute lymphoblastic 108
  acute myeloid 31, 108–9
  chronic granulocytic 31, 32, 107, 109
  chronic lymphocytic 112
  promyelocytic 34, 113
Lewy bodies 46, 141
lignocaine
  ECG effects 15, 70
  sodium conductance and 74
likelihood ratio 65, 183
lipodystrophy, partial 169
lipoprotein lipase deficiency 153
lipoproteins 153
lithium toxicity 87

liver
  enlarged (hepatomegaly) 27, 30–1, 98, 106–7, 109
  metastases 100
  transplantation 102
liver disease, chronic 27, 29, 98, 102–3
liver enzyme tests 52, 153
liver failure, acute 29, 102
*LQT2 HERG* gene 70
*LQT3 SCN5A* gene 70
lung cancer 56, 162
lupus anticoagulant 109
lupus erythematosus, systemic *see* systemic lupus erythematosus
luteinising hormone 86, 92
Lyme disease (*Borrelia burgdorferi* infection) 35, 47, 116, 142
lymphogranuloma venereum 119
lymphoma 34, 113
  gastric MALT 93
  non-Hodgkin's 34, 113

macrophages 33, 112
malabsorption 25, 93–4, 100
malaria 37, 119
  cerebral 120
  falciparum 37, 120
  prophylaxis 35, 116–17
Mann–Whitney $U$ test 65, 181
Marfan's syndrome 79
mathematical medicine 62–6, 173–85
mean
  arithmetical 63, 173
  population vs sample 63, 177
  standard error (SEM) 63, 177
median 62, 173
medullary sponge kidney 131
mefenamic acid 52, 154
mefloquine 35, 116
Meigs' syndrome 55, 161
melanoptysis 159

# Index

membranous nephro-
pathy 40–1, 127
metformin 50, 88, 149
methotrexate 61, 171
metoprolol 40, 124
midbrain lesions 48, 146
middle cerebral artery 43,
134, *135*
migraine 141, 147
milk alkali syndrome 43, 131
minimal change nephropathy 41,
128
minoxidil 40, 124
mitral regurgitation 15, 70
mitral stenosis 17, 75
mode 63, 173
molecular biology 4–5
monoamine oxidase
inhibitors 48–9, 146–7
monocytes 33, 112
mononeuritis multiplex 45–6, 139
motor neurone disease 46, 48,
139, 144
motor neuropathy 140
mucosa associated lymphoid tissue (MALT) lymphoma,
gastric 93
multiple endocrine neoplasia
(MEN) 91, 92
multiple sclerosis 45, 138, 139
muscle
wasting 59, 166
weakness, distal 47, 142–3
weakness, proximal 21, 86
muscular dystrophy,
Duchenne 47, 86, 142
myasthenia gravis 46, 140–1
mycobacteria, atypical 118
mycoplasma infection 31, 107
*Mycoplasma pneumoniae*
infections 58, 164
mycosis fungoides 34, 113
myeloma 32–3, 111, 170
myocardial infarction
anterior 76, 77
cocaine associated 49, 147

heart block in 77
inferior 76, 77
non-Q wave 18, 77–9
secondary prevention 51, 74–5,
77, 151
myopathy
proximal 21, 86
distal 47, 142–3
myxoma, left atrial 45, 137

*N*-acetyl-cysteine 52, 155
*Necator americanus* 38, 121–2
neonates, cyanosis in 16, 72–3
nephrocalcinosis 42–3, 131
nephrology 39–43, 124–34
nephropathy
diabetic 41–2, 88, 128–9
drugs inducing 42, 129
IgA 41, 127
membranous 40–1, 127
minimal change 41, 128
in sickle-cell disease 106
nephrotic syndrome 42, 109, 127,
128, 129–30
neurofibromatosis 91
neurology 43–8, 134–46
nifedipine 51, 124, 151
nitric oxide 50, 148
nitrofurantoin 124
L-N-monomethyl-L-arginine
(L-NMMA) 148
non-Hodgkin's lymph-
oma 34, 113
nonparametric data 64, 65, 181
nonsteroidal anti-inflammatory
drugs (NSAIDs) 61–2,
171–2
gastrointestinal complications
26, 27, 95–7, 99
in gout 50, 150
renal complications 124–5,
171–2
noradrenaline 44, 136
note taking 9–10
NSAIDs *see* nonsteroidal anti-
inflammatory drugs

# Index

octreotide 28, 100
oculo-cephalic (doll's eye) reflex 47–8, 143
odds ratio 64, 178–9
oesophageal acid reflux 29, 101
oesophageal varices 98
oestrogens 53, 83, 91, 156
ondansetron 47, 49, 51, 141, 147, 151
oral contraceptive pill 51, 151
osteoclast activating factor (OAF) 111
osteogenesis imperfecta 80
osteomalacia 62, 172–3
osteomyelitis, salmonella 106
osteoporosis 21, 62, 86, 172
overdose
  paracetemol 52, 154–5
  aspirin 53, 156–7
  digoxin 53, 157
oxygen
  alveolar gas:arterial blood gradient 55, 160
  concentration, arterial 55, 160
  haemoglobin affinity 31, 108

Paget's disease of bone 62, 172
pancreatitis
  acute 25–6, 94
  chronic 97
paracetamol overdose 52, 154–5
parametric data 64, 178
parasitic infections 38, 121–2, 164
  amoebic disease 38, 121
  cryptococcal infection 118, 144
  cryptosporidium 28, 99, 118
  cysticercosis 123
  filariasis 57, 164
  giardiasis 28, 99–100
  hydatid disease 39, 123
  kala azar 36, 117
  leishmaniasis 36, 107, 117
  pneumocystis 51, 151
  schistosomiasis 28, 36, 99, 106–7, 118
  trypanosomiasis 75–6
  worms 38–9, 110, 121–2
parasympathetic nervous system 44, 134–5
parathyroid hormone (PTH) 23, 88–9
parenteral nutrition, total 52, 152–4
parietal cortex lesions 48, 144
Parkinson's disease 46, 141, 152
patent ductus arteriosus 15, 16, 70–1, 72
penicillamine 42, 61, 129, 171
penicillins 53, 155
peptic ulceration 26, 93, 95–7
  in end-stage renal failure 43, 133
  pyloric stenosis complicating 29, 101–2
pericarditis, constrictive 16, 55, 71–2, 98, 160
peripheral nerve thickening 45, 138
peripheral neuropathy, isoniazid induced 51, 151
peripheral resistance 76
peripheral vascular disease 51, 151
peroneal muscular atrophy 142
pethidine 49, 146
phaeochromocytoma 23–4, 91
pharmacology 48–53, 146–57
phenothiazines 87
phenylbutazone 62, 172
phenytoin 53, 105, 157
Philadelphia chromosome 31, 107
phosphate
  renal excretion 39, 124
  in renal failure 89, 133
photosensitivity 53, 155
pigeon fancier's lung 57, 164
pilot studies 65, 182
plantar responses, up-going 46, 139
plasmin 111–12
platelets 50, 74, 149

# Index

pleural effusion 55, 160
*Pneumocystis carinii* infection 51, 151
pneumonia 57, 163
polio 54, 159
polyarteritis
  microscopic 60, 168
  nodosa 57, 139, 164
polychondritis, relapsing 80
polycystic kidney disease 43, 131–3
polycystic ovary syndrome 21, 86
polymerase chain reaction (PCR) 95, *96*
  amplification refractory mutation system (ARMS-PCR) 132–3
polymyalgia rheumatica 59, 166
polymyositis 59, 166
polyuria 21, 87
population 177
porphyria 102–4
  acute intermittent 46, *103*, 104, 139–40
posterior cerebral arteries 43, 134, *135*
potassium
  in cardiac action potential 74
  ECG effects 15–16, 71
  renal excretion 39, 124
power, study 65, 181, 182
predictive value
  negative 65, 182, 183
  positive 65, 182, 183
prednisolone 52, 155
pregnancy
  antihypertensive therapy 51, 151
  folate deficiency 105
  normal changes 24, 92
  serum thyroxine 85
prevalence 183
prion related disease 44, 137
prolactin 87, 92, 93
proportional hazards analysis, Cox's 66, 185

propranolol 51, 151
prospective studies 64, 178–9
protein C deficiency 109
protein S deficiency 109
psittacosis 57, 119, 164
psoriasis 60, 168, 170
pulmonary artery wedge pressure 57, 75, 164
pulmonary eosinophilia 55, 57, 161, 163–4
pulmonary fibrosis 56, 161–2
  progressive massive 54, 159
  upper vs lower zones 56, 162
pulmonary haemosiderosis, idiopathic 57, 163
pulmonary infections, recurrent 55, 161
pulse rate, slow 19, 81
pulsus paradoxus 16, 71–2
pupillary light reflex 47, 143
pupils, dilated 48, 144, 147
Purtscher's angiopathic retinopathy 94
*p* value 65, 180
pyloric stenosis, adult 29, 101
pyridostigmine 51, 152
pyridoxine 151

QTc interval 15, 69–70
  prolonged 15, 70
questions, exam
  core subjects 3
  favourite 3–4
  innovative 4–5
  practising 6–8
  predicting 1–2
  topical subjects 2–3
quinidine 15, 70

randomized controlled trials 65, 181
reflexes, absent leg 46, 139
regression, linear 64, 179–80
regression analysis 64, 179–80
  multiple 64–5, 180
relapsing polychondritis 80

# Index

renal artery stenosis 40, 125–6
renal blood flow, drugs affecting 41, 127
renal failure
  acute, in falciparum malaria 120
  in acute myeloid leukaemia 109
  aspirin in 75
  chronic
    amyloidosis 43, 61, 133, 170
    anaemia 112
    antihypertensive therapy 51, 151
    bone disease 89, 173
    clotting disorders 112
    drug elimination in 40, 124
    drugs inducing 42, 129
    end-stage 43, 133
renal tubular acidosis 42, 130
renal tubular necrosis, acute 87
respiratory function testing 53, 157–8
respiratory medicine 53–8, 157–65
restriction fragment length polymorphism (RFLP) 131–2
retinoic acid receptor alpha (*RARα*) gene 34, 113
retinopathy
  diabetic 88
  Purtscher's angiopathic 94
retrospective studies 64, 65, 178–9, 181–2
revision 9–11
Rhesus incompatibility 34, 114
rheumatoid arthritis 58, 59, 165, 166
  anaemia in 112
  drug treatment 61, 171
  osteoporosis in 86
  pulmonary fibrosis 56, 162
rheumatoid factor 60, 168
rheumatology 58–62, 165–73
rifampicin 38, 51, 122, 151
right bundle branch block 15, 70

risk, relative 64, 178–9
risk factors 64, 178–9
Romano–Ward syndrome 15, 70
round worms 38, 121

salbutamol
  action 19, 52, 82, 154
  and atenolol 51, 152
  potassium wasting 52, 155
*Salmonella typhi* infections 37, 120
sample 177
sarcoidosis
  broncho-alveolar lavage lymphocytes 57, 163
  cerebrospinal fluid lymphocytes 48, 144
  diagnosis 54, 158–9
  nephrocalcinosis in 43, 131
  respiratory features 53, 56, 157, 162
scattergram 65, 181
Schirmer's test 59, 166
schistosomiasis 28, 36, 99, 106–7, 118
sciatic nerve stretch test 59, 167
scleroderma (systemic sclerosis) 56, 101, 161
secretin 25
selegiline 49, 146–7
sensitivity 65, 182
sensory neuropathy 46, 139–40
seronegative arthritides 61, 80, 170–1
serotonin (5 hydroxytryptamine) 47, 49, 141, 147
Sézary syndrome 34, 113
sickle-cell disease 30, 106
sick sinus syndrome 81
single stranded conformational polymorphism (SSCP) 132
sinus dysrhythmia 15, 69
Sjögren's syndrome 59, 60, 166, 169
skin, reactions to drugs 53, 155–6
sleep apnoea 58, 165

# Index

small bowel ulcers 27, 99
sodium
   in cardiac action potential 74
   excretion 39, 76, 124
specificity 65, 182
spinal cord
   dorsal columns 45, 138–9
   subacute combined degeneration 138–9
   termination 44, 134
splenomegaly 30–1, 106–7, 109
standard deviation 63, 173, 174–6
standard error of mean (SEM) 63, 177
staphylococcal food poisoning 38, 123
steatorrhoea 93
steroids
   biosynthesis 83, *84*
   metabolism 20, 83
   *see also* corticosteroids
streptococcal infections 38, 122–3
streptomycin 38, 122
stroke 44, 48, 136, 144–6
   risk factors 45, 137
*Strongyloides stercoralis* 38, 122
Student's *t* test 64, 178
sulphonamides 53, 155
sulphonylureas 50, 84, 88, 149
sumatriptan 47, 49, 141, 147
supraventricular tachycardia 18, 49, 79–80, 148
survival analysis 66, 183–5
sympathetic nervous system 134–6
syphilis 48, 79, 80, 138, 144
systemic lupus erythematosus 58, 59, 165–6
   antibodies in 60, 169
   diffuse alveolar haemorrhage 57, 163
   hypocomplementaemia 60, 169
systemic sclerosis (scleroderma) 56, 101, 161

tabes dorsalis 138
tachycardia
   supraventricular 18, 49, 79–80, 148
   ventricular 18, 79–80
*Taenia solium* 39, 123
T cell development 33, 112
temporal arteritis 59, 60, 166, 167
temporal lobe lesions 48, 144
testicular feminization syndrome 22, 87
testosterone 83, 87
tetanus 34–5, 114–15
thalassaemia 106, 108, 110
thiamine *see* vitamin $B_1$
threadworms 38, 121
thrombocytopaenia 30, 105
thrombophilia, systemic 32, 109
thymoma 46, 140
thyroid cancer 24, 92
thyroiditis 85
thyroid stimulating hormone (TSH) 85
thyrotoxicosis (hyperthyroidism) 20–1, 85, 86
thyrotrophin-releasing hormone (TRH) 85
thyroxine (T4), serum 85
tolbutamide 50, 149
toxocara infection 35–6, 117
transfusion, blood 34, 113–14
transketolase, red cell 47, 107
tretinoin 34, 113
triamcinolone 52, 155
triamterene 51, 151–2
*Trichuris trichuria* 38, 122
tricyclic antidepressants 47, 49, 141, 146
triiodothyronine (T3), serum 85
*Trypanosoma cruzi* infection 75–6
*t* test 64, 178
tuberculosis 54, 118, 158
   cerebrospinal fluid lymphocytes 48, 144
   drug therapy 38, 122
   pleural effusion 55, 160

# Index

tuberculosis *(Cont.)*
  spinal 167
Turner's syndrome 92–3
typhoid fever 37, 120
tyramine 49, 146

ulcerative colitis 27, 98, 100
unconscious patient 47–8, 143–4
urea 39, 124
urinary tract infection (UTI) 40, 125
urine, acid 101
ursodeoxycholic acid 98, 100

vanillylmandelic acid (VMA) 91
variance 63, 175
varicella zoster infection 37, 119
vasoactive intestinal peptide (VIP) 25, 94
ventilation : perfusion ratio 55, 160
ventilation, increased 55, 160
ventricular septal defect 16, 56, 72, 162
ventricular tachycardia 18, 79–80
verapamil 49, 82, 148
vertebral arteries 134, *135*
villous atrophy, partial 28, 99
vincristine 51, 150
visual pathway 144, *145*
vitamin $B_1$ (thiamine) 51, 151
  deficiency 47, 94, 107, 141–2
vitamin $B_{12}$
  deficiency 44, 46, 104, 136, 138–9, 140
  high levels 31, 107
vitamin D
  deficiency 59, 86, 93, 166, 172–3
  sythesis 89, *90*
vitamin K deficiency 93–4
vomiting, drug induced 51, 151
von Willebrand factor 50, 149
von Willebrand's disease 105, 111

Waldenstrom's macroglobulinaemia 59, 166
warfarin
  drug interactions 30, 105
  in stroke prevention 44, 136
water excretion 39, 124
Wegener's granulomatosis 57, 163, 168
Wernicke–Korsakoff's syndrome 142
Whipple's disease 28, 97, 99
whipworms 38, 122
white cell antigen reactions 34, 114
Widal test 120
Wilson's disease 47, 143
Wolff–Parkinson–White syndrome 19, 81–2
worms 38, 121–2
writing materials 11

*Yersinia* infections 28, 99

Zollinger–Ellison syndrome 26, 97